MW01615874

ANTI-CANCER
HABITS & ANTI-INFLAMMATORY NUTRITION

HOLISTIC HEALTH
LILLY PADILLA

Design and layout by Nicole Leibman.

Library of Congress Cataloging-In-Publication Data available.

ISBN 10: 0692445862
ISBN 13: 978-0-692-44586-0

Printed in the United States of America

www.lillypadilla.com

May this book be an inspiration to those looking to prevent cancer, inflammatory diseases, and avoid recurrences of cancer. May they find balance and harmony by nourishing their body with the energy of nutritional whole foods and a holistic approach to life.

TABLE OF CONTENTS

Chapter 4: Managing Stress

Chapter 5: Digestion and Cancer

Lilly's Recipes

Eating with a Purpose in Mind

Conclusion

Forming Habits and Adapting to Better Health

Aknowlodgements and Bibliography

chapter 1

MY STORY

"The first wealth is health"

- Ralph Waldo Emerson

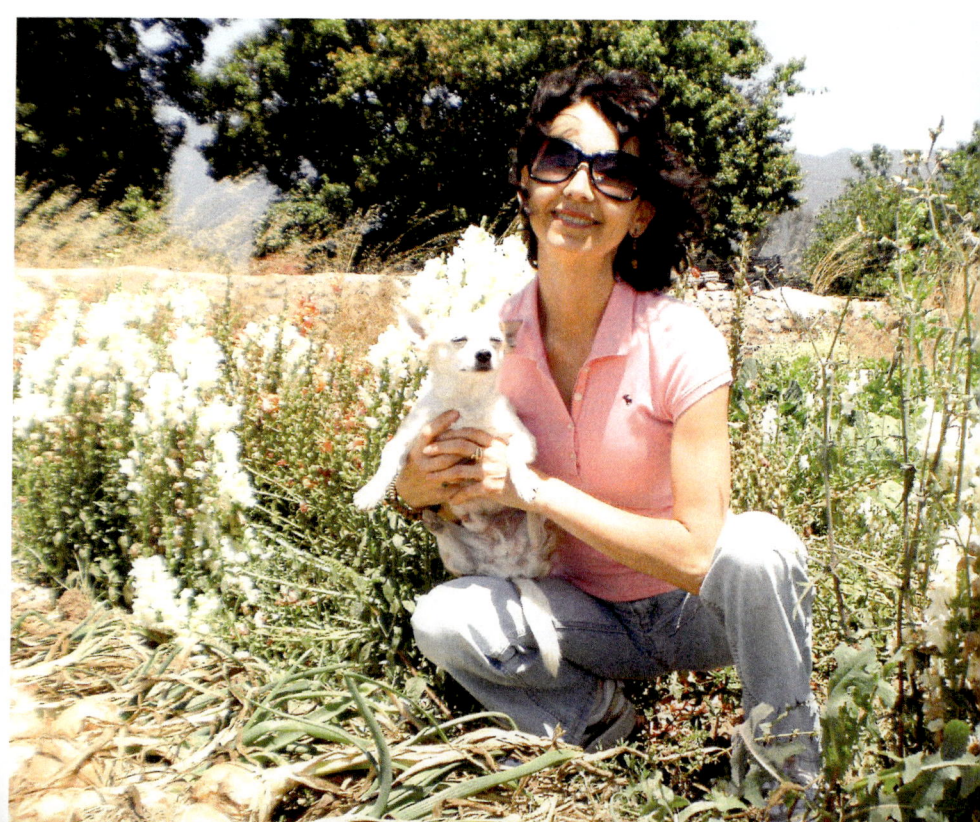

Is Illness a Door for Transformation?

Twelve years ago, after many visits to the doctors, and months of persistence, I realized they were not sure what was happening to my body. I had to insist and pressure them to give me an ultrasound, a CT scan and a refferal to a specialist. I was not feeling well for months. Finally, they sent me to see the head of the cancer department at a well known hospital in Los Angeles. The surgeon Gynocological oncologist did a thorough vaginal exam and said: "You don't have anything, it is only a 0.2% chance of being cancer. I'm going on vacation and I will see you again when I come back in a few weeks". I remember that my sister Diana (who is a nurse anesthetist) was with me and we were so relieved and happy with the news from the doctor. A few hours later however, the symptoms for which I sought medical advice (abdominal bloating, cramping, uncomfortable feeling in the lower abdomen, unstable digestion, dull mind, inability to sleep, and craving sugary foods every day) were back again. Two days later the symptoms got even worse; I was having heavy bleeding outside of my period, felt horribly bloated, and was experiencing profound sadness. On top of everything, I started rapidly losing weight. I knew something was wrong.

By the time the oncologist came back from his vacation I was in terrible pain, very weak, overly bloated,

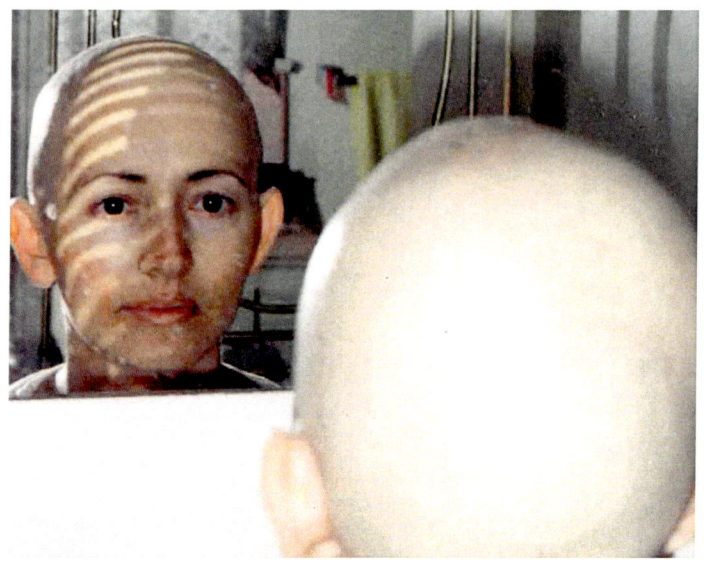

was not able to eat. I had to have a rushed laparoscopy surgery. I remember that a few minutes before the surgery, the surgeon asked me, "If I see that it is cancer, may I take everything out?" It meant I wouldn't be able to have children, and the possibility of having cancer. Instead of a short laparoscopy, the surgery took many hours and the tumor was so big it broke apart as he tried to pull it out. When I woke up from the surgery, I remember seeing my mother crying. I knew then - it was ovarian cancer.

My first reaction was: Why me? Where did I go wrong? What can I do to help my body? At the time I didn't make the connection, I didn't know of the severe damage that one can do to the body with toxic foods, toxic relationships, too much stressful thinking, and negative emotions. It all contributes to the sickness or wellness of the cells. Now I monitor not only my eating, but also my sleep, moods, energy level, stress level and social interactions.

After the diagnosis and during the treatments, my goal was to learn to understand my body, to be proactive and to not focus on cancer. I **focused on wellness**, nutrition and research on both nutritional scientific findings and Chinese Nutritional Therapy. My main purpose was, and still is today, to create healthy, happy cells.

I actually started calling myself a cancer survivor right after surgery, since I survived the surgery, chemo and radiation. The rest was, and still is, up to me. Holistic Nutrition has been the door for transforming my cells into happy healthy cells. It is an ongoing process; from shopping for groceries for nutritional cooking, to creating the right healthy habits for my life and focusing on nurturing my cells, body and mind.

Cancer opened up a door for curiosity, learning and understanding both western medicine and Eastern Traditional Chinese Medicine and its unique Chinese

Nutritional Therapy, which led me to fall in love with holistic nutrition. At the beginning it was for my own nutritional needs, cooking and eating habits. I went from a bad experience and feeling depressed to having a wonderful job and finding my purpose in life. Fortunately, my passion for nutrition grew so much I went back to school and ended up changing careers. I became a Certified Integrative Nutrition Health Coach and Nutritional chef. I am lucky that I'm able to help the community be healthier, and do what I love to do the most.

Being Our Own Health Advocates

Now after 12 years of transformation and learning nutrition, I can make a clear connection between what happened to me and what I did to my body. No one is responsible for my health but me. It is a priority to be an advocate for my health and wellness, I'm eternally grateful for the opportunity to change my life and prioritize my health, nutrition and wellness. Doctors are there to help us, but it is our responsibility to take care of our body and mind. *Nobody knows your body better than you.* Listening to your body's signs and symptoms is being in touch with yourself. The communication with doctors and health professionals needs be open and clear for them to help you understand what is happening in your body. However, they can only guide you, real healing comes from within you. It is your body and your mind, be proactive in managing your health, be your own health advocate, listen and follow your body signs and intuition.

Starving Cancer Cells

Starving cancer cells became my goal. How? I armed myself with the tools from the very essence of life, understanding where and how energy is born. I went back to the books to learn the basics of biology, physiology, soil, food, and the influence of natural laws from the Traditional Chinese Medicine perspective, one of the oldest medicines in the planet, along with Ayurveda. One unique concept both medicines agree on is the five flavors, and five elements of the earth. The five flavors are: sweet, sour, pungent, bitter and salty. Unfortunately, in America, the SAD (Standard American Diet) diet is mainly based on things that are sweet and salty, missing the value and chemistry of the other not so common flavors: sour, pungent, and bitter. Each flavor provides us with some specific chemistry that helps us maintain balance in the body. It is so beautiful to learn to manage the five flavors and realize that they have a deep connection with the five elements and our five senses (smell, taste, sight, touch and sound). I will be discussing the properties of the five flavors more in depth in the following chapters. Come along! Let's be healthy!

chapter 2

INFLAMMATION

"Symptoms, then are in reality nothing but the cry from suffering organs"

- Jean Martin Charcot

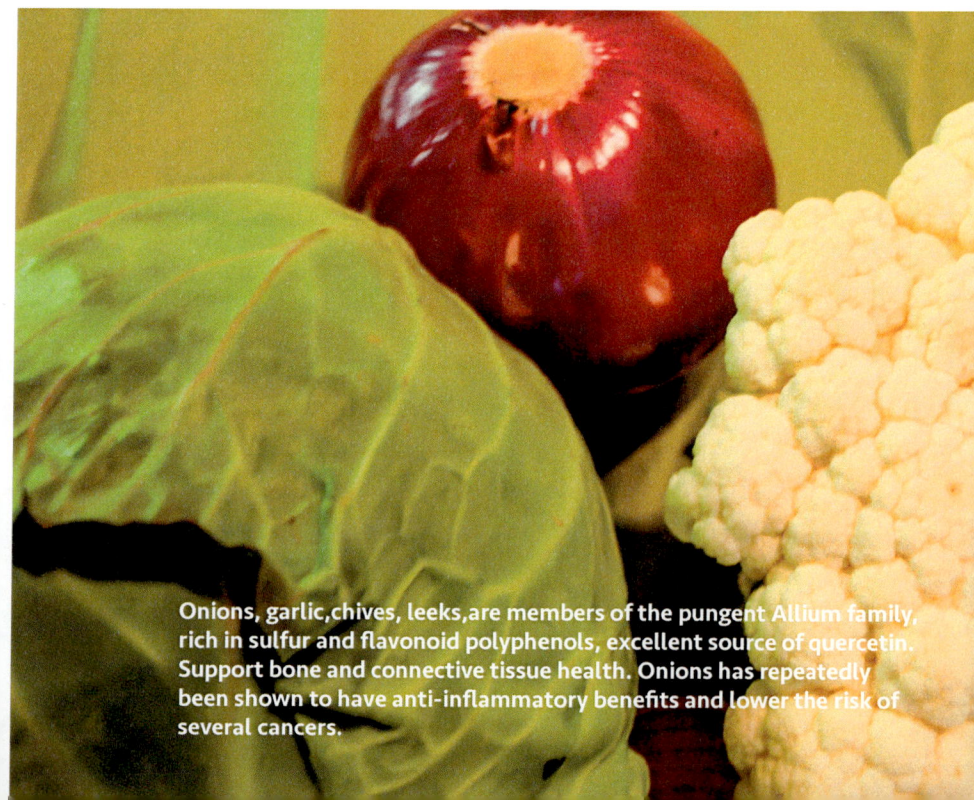

Onions, garlic,chives, leeks,are members of the pungent Allium family, rich in sulfur and flavonoid polyphenols, excellent source of quercetin. Support bone and connective tissue health. Onions has repeatedly been shown to have anti-inflammatory benefits and lower the risk of several cancers.

What is Inflammation?

Inflammation is an immune response to injury, toxins, allergies, or infections. It is set up to protect the body. Many studies have shown that toxin build up in the body can cause acidification of the blood pH and over time will promote or cause chronic inflammation.

I can't discuss the subject of inflammation and cancer without explaining what acidification is and how it leads to chronic inflammation. When I refer to acidification, I'm referring to blood pH acidification. It is important to learn about acidic blood pH because it's a major precursor to chronic inflammation in the body.

Blood pH is the acidity or alkalinity of blood. I call it , in a holistic way, **P**ure **H**armony, for it is the center point for keeping the body in balanced harmony, just like the yin and yang balances the body as well. In biology, the pH of any fluid is the measure of the hydrogen ion (H+) concentration. The lower the pH, the more acidic the blood will become.

In 2003, when I was diagnosed with ovarian cancer, I had many of the symptoms of acidic pH. Nowadays, observing and talking to clients with cancer and other inflammatory diseases, I've noticed that they all have something in common. A big percentage of them presented symptoms of acidic blood pH before getting diagnosed. A healthy body operates in a narrow pH range, should be slightly more alkaline than acidic, around a range 7.365. Even just a pinch more acidic than alkaline ranges can create disasters in all the system's functions and rhythmic patterns of the body, leading to inflammatory diseases.

Chronic inflammation is responsible for many diseases, including heart disease, metabolic syndrome, arthritis, lupus, Intestinal Bowel Syndrome (IBS), cancer, diabetes, and even Alzheimer's. Systematic inflammation is a key factor in neurodegeneration.

Research shows that there is usually a period of blood acidification before chronic inflammation occurs. Imagine this picture: *if I pour acid over my hand it will create an inflammatory response. I will experience pain, redness, heat, and swelling in the affected area.* Imagine your acidic blood causing a similar inflammatory response like heat, swelling, and pain along your body, which, if left unchecked for a long period of time, will develop into chronic inflammation. Furthermore, many studies indicate when chronic inflammation goes unchecked, it appears to increase tumor development.

Where Does Acidic Blood pH Come From?

We create new cells every single day with the nutrients from the food that we put in our mouth. Food is chemistry, and we are made out of pure chemistry in balance. The body is a unique process in motion, making healthy or unhealthy cells according to its chemistry, which is the outcome of our nutrition and lifestyle.

Most babies come into this world as happy and healthy humans who are full of energy! And of course they have normal blood pH. Over the years, we can easily get out of our balanced chemistry or blueprint as we consume the wrong food, too much sugar or salt, (or any food flavor in extreme), foods with chemicals, or modified foods that rapidly can change the chemistry of our bodies. Literally we become what we eat, changing the body's chemistry constantly, which is easily observed when we take a blood panel. One day the numbers can be normal, the next day it may be out of range. We do have the power to alter our chemistry every single time we eat.

There are acid forming foods and alkaline forming foods. Having a balanced diet that combines more alkaline than acid forming foods is the best way to enhance longevity and good health. The problem arises when we intake large amounts of acid forming foods, which contribute to the creation of acidic blood pH.

Just like anything else on the planet, we are a part of the process of life. We are a process in motion, which means our bodies are a unit of processes. For us to become new everyday we go through a process; we eat, breathe, create energy, use energy, eliminate waste and renew ourselves as we sleep and rest. Each of these stages is a process in itself. In the process of inflammation, there is a slightly acidic blood pH in the cells of every single tissue of our bodies. Specifically, the *interstitial space* around the cell becomes acidic, damaging the cells, so as the result they might become sick, mutate or die because of the acid in the interstitial space. **The acids are killing the tissues that make up every single organ in our bodies**. The organs can't function well, and this affects body processes and natural biorhythms, making us feel out of balance. Hence sickness shows up.

Common examples of inflamed tissues in the body include: burning stomach sensation, bleeding gums, gingivitis, tender joints, IBS, arthritis, osteoarthritis, lupus, multiple sclerosis, ulcers, allergies, itchy rash, swollen wrist and feet, asthma. These are just some examples of extreme inflammations in the body that start with high acidic blood pH.

There are many things that can spike acidic pH,

including: what we eat, how we eat, what we do on a daily basis, our stress level, and what we don't do (like the habit of not exercising). Lack of exercise contributes to the acidification process. Remember, we are a process in motion, which is why moderate movement promotes the functioning and synchronicity of our body's processes. Exercise also promotes oxygen intake and release of toxins, reinforcing the healing processes within the body. Stillness and rigidity hold acids and toxins in, promoting acidic blood pH. On the other hand, excessive or extreme exercise can have a negative effect by adding more acid to the body. There it is again, the yin-yang synergy in the body. Anything in extremes can pull the balance out of our yin-yang center (which, in biological terms, is our pH level). Hence, avoiding going into extremes is key to preserving balance. On the next page you can find Doctor Yang-chu Higgins' traditional chinese medicine perspective on balance and our health.

☯

The Five Flavors: According to TCM, **excess** use of any of the five flavors affects our chemistry causing imbalances. One common example of excess is **sweet flavor-sugars**, which contribute to acidic blood pH, and inflammatory diseases like diabetes and **cancer**. **Salty** is the other overly consumed flavor in modern society. Both of these flavors when consumed in excess may contribute to cancer cell proliferation. Adding the other flavors: pungent, sour and bitter helps control the cravings for sweet and salty foods.

A Traditional Chinese Medicine Perspective on Imbalances

by Yang-chu Higgins, LAc, EFT-Adv

Lilly was kind enough to ask me to write on the subject of inflammation from a Chinese medical perspective. For starters, it is important to understand that terms like "inflammation" do not exist in traditional Chinese medicine. What there is is a set of conditions that manifest as a result of either external or internal influences called "pathogens" or xie qi. In all likelihood it is the presence of these pathogenic factors that lead to what is called inflammation, but from this perspective inflammation is only the result of that which is caused by pathogens. This may seem like a purely technical matter, but it is not, for treatment strategies are devised around the nature of the pathogen, i.e., the cause, and not its effect. In short, pathogens are treated not inflammation. Below, a brief discussion of what constitutes a pathogen in Chinese medicine will hopefully clarify this important if subtle distinction.

A "pathogen" is an agent that upsets the body's balance. It can come from outside the body invading by way of wind, thus affecting the lungs and upper part of the body or be ingested, affecting the stomach and digestive system. Internal pathogens arise from some malfunction of an organ system. Underlying weakness an organ, while not in itself pathogenic, can allow pathogens to gain a foothold in the body. **These weaknesses may arise as a course of lifestyle, work, diet, or genetic influences.**

Pathogens to the Western mind are nearly universally associated with bacteria and viruses. These influences are mostly identified as "wind" in Chinese medicine. In fact, within the Chinese character for wind is an element that denotes bug, worms or other creepy-crawlies. By Chinese medicine reckoning these bugs endeavor to drive as deeply into the body as the immune system will allow, the heart being the endgame. Whether this is clinically true or not, there can be no mistake that exterior pathogens play a critical role in creating imbalance in the body dynamics which could be construed as having some bearing on inflammation. Long-term residence of external pathogens will invariably weaken body function, giving rise to a breakdown of the overall system, with pathology expressed in multiple physiological systems

"Wei qi" is a Chinese medical term that describes the body's ability to fend off exterior attacks. It might be a term referring to humoral immunity, as wei qi is mostly connected with the lungs. When the wei qi is unable to protect the body and the pathogen takes up residence in one of the systems of the body, energy is constantly allocated to try to rid the body of the invader. If the pathogen is not eliminated, the body will continue to fight, at the expense of other normal physiological activity. This is how the cascade of imbalance occurs, since there is only so much energy overall that the body has to allocate.

Critically, wei qi deficiency is the inability of the body to muster the strength to fight and defend at the level of the lung. Deficiency could be characterized as the lack of fire necessary to kill invaders. This is to say **inflammation that arises as a result of the immune response is key in rooting out colonizing pathogens.**

The objective in holisitic nutrition is to provide instruction onto how to fit foods into a strategy of fighting pathogenic factors using the comprehensive system of Chinese medicine. There are many varying schools of thought regarding the ideal diet. The art and advantage of Chinese medicine is that universal prescriptions are forgone in favor of a tailored approach based on each individual's presentation.

Many dietary trends tend to appear on their face to be common sense and healthful. Take the suggestion of eating five servings of fruit and five servings of vegetables daily. This should be fairly helpful advice to follow but is it really? The guidelines, for example, are unclear about whether the vegetables should be cooked or raw and assume that there are no pre-existing conditions that would make consumption of so much sugar, albeit natural, prudent.

Chinese medicine sees a clear difference between the natures of cooked and raw food that has direct implications for how the body will metabolize that which is consumed. The vitalizing aspects of fruit cannot be made use of when digestion is not strong and influenced by dysbiosis, that is conditions like yeast and imbalanced gut flora. The underlying constitution of foods and their preparation cannot be over emphasized.

There is also a prevailing trend born from nutrition "science" that seeks to break food down into theoretical components with the presumption being that parts is parts: that is to say one part this component is the equivalent to one part that part component. These components are commonly known as proteins, fats, fiber, vitamins and minerals. A true holistic approach to food, which Chinese medicine takes, axiomatically rejects this perspective. **Whole food is more than the sum of its parts**. Frozen or reconstituted food is not the same as that which is fresh from the garden. Proteins of this sort are not only equivalent to proteins of that sort, but also the very notion of reductionist claims about proteins and the like.

Instead of viewing food within the confines of nutritionism, all food is viewed as having a particular constitution that conforms to the overall system of Chinese medicine.   The key is the signs that the body elicits in terms of energy, tongue picture, and pulse. These signs show metabolism, pathological status, and strength of the body. There are numerous permutations to how food can be interpreted using the tools of modern science. Some have more validity than others, though they are not conclusive. There are plenty of vegetarians, for example who contract cancer and there are smokers who often live into their 80s. It is simply not possible to reduce health to any one factor. But by knowing how to read the signs that your body exhibits you can go far in bringing a healthful balance to your body using the comprehensive system that is offered by Chinese medicine.

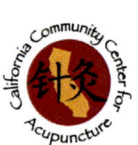

Yang-chu Higgins, LAc, EFT-Adv is an acupuncturist and herbalist since 2008. He has studied Chinese at Peking university and possesses a master's degree from U Michigan's Center for Chinese Studies. He has successfully treated conditions ranging from insomnia to chronic fatigue, migraines to debilitating arthritis. His focus is on treating functional aspects of chronic conditions, including those related to fertility. His website is http://ccc-a.us. Phone number: 323.936.5152.

How We Eat, What We Eat, and How We Prepare Food

According to Traditional Chinese Medicine and nutritional therapy teachings, there are levels of acid forming foods and alkaline forming foods. This is not a new concept in nutrition. For thousands of years, oriental traditions have used the properties of food to preserve balanced pH levels. These traditions consider the thermal nature of the food (heating, cooling, or warming), the five tastes or flavors (sweet, bitter, salty, sour, pungent) and the acid-alkaline nature of the foods. In fact, many dishes are created with these concepts, plus the seasonal attunement in mind, to help a person come back into balance, just like I did. In respect to acid-alkaline foods, many oriental cultures have used an easy approach to eating for thousands of years. They eat more fresh vegetables and produce than animal meats and dairy products. Let's see how this works.

Between the acid forming foods, all meats, dairy and especially cheese are highly acidic. Some grains and beans can contribute to the formation of acid as well, since they carry waste within their skin that can create bits of acidification. But grains and beans have a mild acid forming effect compared to that of animal foods. These grains, beans, and even seeds have a mid to low range of acidification, and this varies based on how they are soaked, prepared, and ingested. Sprouted beans,

Sprouts *are full of energy! They represent the point of greatest vitality in the life cycle of a plant. We experience this* **energy** *and* **vitality** *when eating sprouts consistently. The process of germination neutralizes phytic acid, which inhibits absorption of many minerals.*

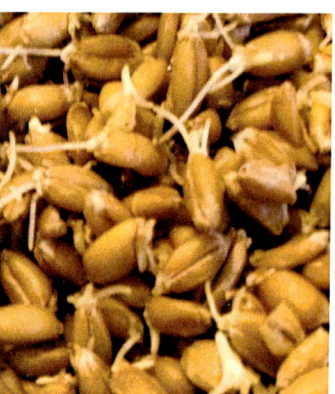 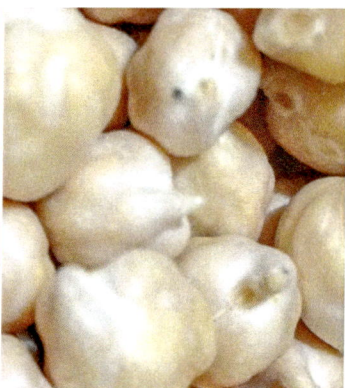 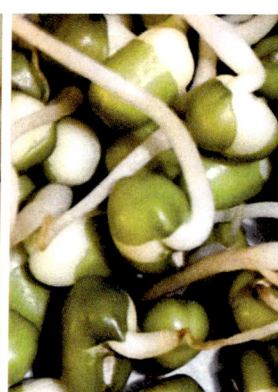

grains, nuts and seeds are much healthier and easier to digest and have a significant increase in nutritional value. *When sprouting beans, grains and seeds we neutralize the enzyme inhibitors, phytic acids, and lectins.* Hence they become less acid forming.

Grains, beans and seeds are more alkaline forming foods once they are sprouted, like a new baby food full of energy and life! They are ready for optimal absorption, helping our digestive system do its work smoothly, and helping us save energy at the same time. Think about it, when we soak a bean or grain, it loosens up the dirty foam and waste like dirt. This is called the "garbage of the grain", and it doesn't belong in the body. So, when we don't soak the grains or the beans, we are putting a little bit more of acid-waste in small amounts and in this way we are contributing to acidification in our bodies. Waste and toxins are the major causes of acidic conditions. Also, most locals in China and India, when cooking non-sprouted beans and grains, remove the layer of foam on top of the water as the beans and grains start boiling. It is best to remove that dirty foam to avoid gas and heavy digestion from non-sprouted beans and grains. There are easy steps to make plant-based proteins easier to digest and to avoid even low acid-forming waste. I can't say the same for animal proteins, which are highly acid-forming. Except for lower ng the intake of them, cooking them in soups, or avoiding them completely if that is your preference.

Dairy, milk and cheese are known to create big amounts of mucus and acidification, so are red meat and any other animal proteins – we cannot soak these foods and sprout them like we do with beans and grains. This is yet another reason why the consumption of animal products can be tricky for certain inflammatory diseases, e.g. arthritis, diabetes, cancer. When there is arthritis, it is well known that red meat makes the inflammation worse. We have a better option when we have plant-based proteins than when we eat animal protein three times a day, like eating the Standard

American Diet (SAD). In reality not everybody needs to have such big amounts of protein. It all depends on the individual, since everybody has different needs according to their age, gender, activity level, work, chemistry, and energy. For example, a 70 year old person that is retired probably doesn't need the same amount of protein than a 14 year old that plays football 5 days a week. The activity level and muscle use require different amounts of protein. *No one diet works for everyone.*

In my case, after cancer, it was important to start minimizing animal products little by little in order to avoid inflammation. By doing this, I allowed new digestion for beans and grains to take place smoothly, creating a new process in the digestion, allowing enzymes to be developed for such foods. Turning to a plant-based diet, which is rich in vitamins, minerals, healthy carbs and proteins, has helped me develop a much healthier energy. But, even within the plant-based diet, I still soak my bean proteins, grains and carbs. Also, I make sure to eat the cleanest and the least inflammatory or acid forming foods that I can. Keeping it simple, by having more vegetables than solid proteins, works for me.

Chronic Inflammation

In his research, Dr. Marti Bosch, an Oncologist from Spain, explains how cells can become sick from too much acid in the interstitial space of the cell. According to his findings, the acid in the interstitial space of the cell burns or damages the area to the point that the cells can't take it anymore and may mutate or die. Also, a long time ago, the Austrian physician Dr. Pischinger wrote about how the integrity of the interstitial system is the most important prerequisite for healthy tissue regulation. He also remarked that some elements can disturb the delicate balance within the interstitial space of the cells like, the protein content, the acid-base balance, and the mineral and trace element content. It is all about maintaining the delicate pH balance within range. Over time, the **accumulation of acids** within the interstitial space can develop into inflammation, which overtime, as accumulation happens, may transform into **chronic inflammation**, dead cells, or mutating cells,

Basic Pischinger System

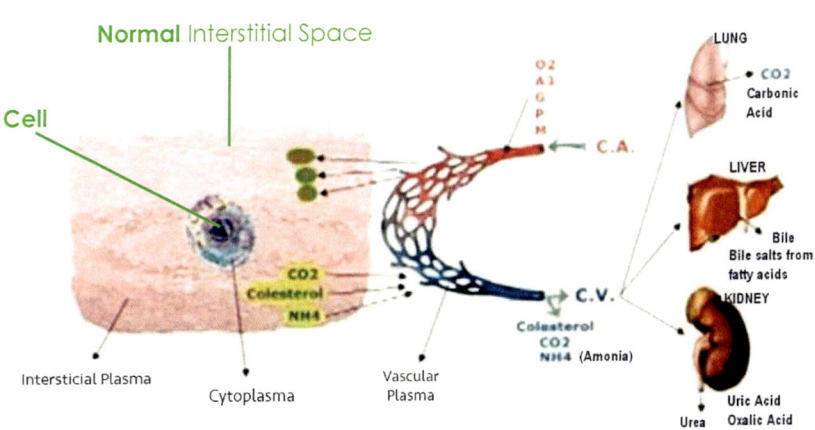

From Dr. Alberto Marti Bosch's Seminar

Basic Pischinger System

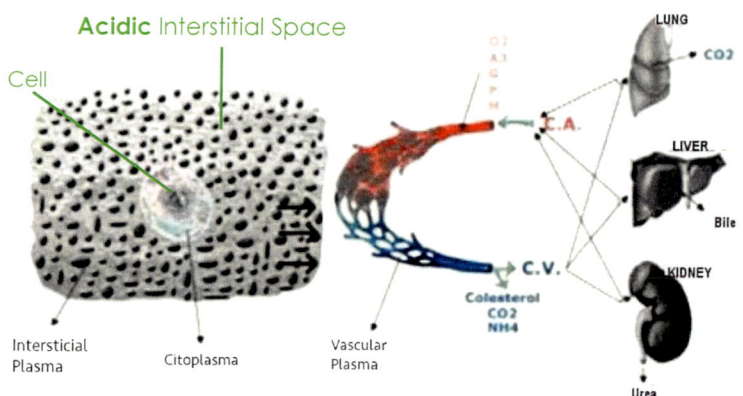

From Dr. Alberto Marti Bosch's Seminar

and **may cause cancer**. In general, it has been shown that every chronically ill person exhibits an imbalance of the inner interstitial space of the cells. Most chronic diseases, such as cancer, arthritis, diabetes, Alzheimer's, heart disease, etc. reflect a similar path: acidification, long term inflammatory response, and then prompt formation of the chronic disease.

It seems many European and American cancer experts agree on one thing: cancer is the inability of cells to die. Meaning those cells probably mutate because they resist dying or can't die because we keep feeding them with the wrong foods. Hence, it would probably be wise to avoid acidic pH and inflammation to avoid these kinds of mutating cells.

For years now, I have been looking at how my body pH and my clients' bodies change when we change the foods we eat in a consistent manner. *Sending the right message to the cells using the right foods is crucial.* So I create my recipes with food synergy in mind. My goal is to send the right message consistently to each cell.

Food makes up our chemistry and energy every day. The more we use green, alkalizing anti-inflammatory meals, organic green soups, green vegetable smoothies, colorful organic salads, and colorful veggie stews, the more we notice our bodies exhibiting greater energy, deeper sleep, a sharper mind, and most importantly, overall good health. I know that, even during and after the cancer diagnosis, my body responded with ease after I changed my diet to whole, pure organic foods with large amounts of vegetables, which helped alkalize the body quickly. Minimizing toxicity, and alkalizing my body has been a priority to maintain good health. *See my recipes in the last chapter!*

As Dr. Pischinger mentioned in his work, we need a diet and lifestyle that supports, nurtures, and detoxifies all cells and tissues by supplying them with needed substances, such as oxygen and nutrients, and by removing cellular waste products and toxins. Hence, we need to move energies and toxins out consistently in order to preserve the health of our bodies.

What organs filter toxins and wastes? Waste is

filtered out of the blood mainly by the liver, kidneys, and lungs, our body filters, along with the skin. We are able to change the filters of our car, our house, our office, but what about the ones of our body? We can not change them. What can we do? We can clean them! What do you use to clean things? Water, plus something to scrub with, right? The process of cleaning our body is similar. We need to eat lots of cleansing vegetables (specially leafy greens), and fiber foods like grains, beans and some fruits to bring down the wastes and toxins. Green Vegetables contain large amounts of water, and are loaded with fiber, chlorophyll micronutrients and phytochemicals.

In Chinese medicine green is associated with the liver. Green vegetables are used for renewal and purification of the blood, and vital energy. Leafy greens are also high-alkaline foods because they also contain good amounts of minerals. We frequently hear that cleansing the liver is important for healthy cells. I agree a hundred percent. The liver is the gate keeper, it performs hundreds of tasks 24 hours a day and 365 days a year to keep our blood healthy. As a major filter, it is in charge of cleansing and purifying the blood. If the blood is clean and pure every day, our cells will be healthier. The opposite is also true, when the liver rhythmic work slows down, there will be an accumulation of toxins. It will also slow down the work of other filters in our bodies. The detoxification process is rhythmic, and it works like a domino effect. The filters are all connected - they work as whole. In TCM, the liver is known to work along with kidneys as a team. When one of the filters is sick or has slowed down from too much work, the other gets a part of that work, but it will slow down the whole process of detoxification. This is when the person might feel slow, heavy, sluggish in many ways reflecting the state of the body filters.

There are other factors that can cause acidic blood. Many of them are related to high stress levels, anxiety, insomnia, poor sleeping patterns, and of course high cortisol levels. I can tell you that before I was diagnosed with cancer I had one of the worst years of stress, sleeplessness, lack of exercise (from too many hours sitting in front of the computer), and a poor diet that consisted mostly of eating convenient, quick meals made with modified ingredients like soy, corn and unhealthy oils.

Other factors that influence acidic blood pH:
- Poor digestion that creates a constant immune response
- Toxin build up such as: carbon dioxide, cholesterol, uric acid, waste from medication
- Tooth infections creating acidic conditions in the mouth

- Emotional stress, mental stress, which produces high cortisol
- Low oxygen intake which influences cellular acidification
- Lack of movement- exercise, stagnancy of the blood or slow flow
- Hidden infections, bacteria, yeast and fungus overgrowth and its toxic waste
- Low nutrients such as minerals, which are needed to counteract acids
- Cumulative toxic effect slowing down body filters (liver, kidneys, lungs)
- Eating high acid forming foods that creates acidic build up

Acidic conditions in the body are like nests for bacteria, yeast and fungi to proliferate. In fact, many common infections are actually caused by bacteria that is already present in the normal flora of our system. But when our diet becomes more acidic, the acid creates the perfect ground for these unfriendly guys to proliferate out of control, resulting in things such as frequent yeast infections, which are known as candida. We are not alone, we are sharing our bodies with millions of bacteria and fungi. Did you know that we have ten times more bacteria than cells in our body? *So we are better off learning how to maintain them under control and live in harmony with them.*

Yeast, Acidification and Cancer

It was winter of 2002 when I first noticed signs that something was changing in my body. The first rashes kept coming back to my body as red patches showed here and there. But the worst was a big itching patch on my leg. It was very rare and since it kept coming back, I decided to show it to my sister, who is a nurse. She thought it was a fungi according to the symptoms.

Weeks went by and other symptoms also showed up. I couldn't sleep well, was irritable, my thinking was very dull, I couldn't focus well, had many yeast infections, and a general lack of energy. I couldn't function normally as I usually would do. I was definitely not myself. *Watch out when you feel uncomfortable, out of balance, and not like your usual self for a period of time. The body is definitely sending signals.*

Within a few weeks, I had other symptoms: abdominal bloating started being noticeable and some bleeding that was happening before and after my period. I was worried. I went to the doctor, briefly mentioned the rashes and itching, but since the focus was on the bleeding only, there was no test for the fungus or yeast. Lots of doctors' appointments followed, as they were trying to find out what was happening.

For sure, eating lots of white yeasted breads and processed foods didn't help me. Once I started educating myself on health and nutrition in both eastern and western approaches to health, I was able to link things together, turn my diet around and finally help my body. I was experiencing yeast infections, itchy rashes, a dull mind, yeast overgrowth and low immunity. I had candida overgrowth before cancer. It started small, but once I was eating too much white bread, had high stress levels, craved sweets, and did not sleep well, candida took over. It sped up and overgrew to the point of lowering my immunity, giving cancer cells the open door to grow. I find that many authors write about it, European doctors, American integrative doctors, several studies nowadays. Also, both Traditional Chinese Medicine (TCM) and Ayurveda have openly connected candida overgrowth with low immunity for hundreds of years.

TCM states that yeast when overgrown many times passes from the intestinal wall into the blood stream and from that point wrecks havoc, inhibiting immunity. Giving a push to acidic conditions in the body, the perfect nesting environment for cancer cells to grow. Candida is a cumulative process that may take months to fully develop, it may depend on the type of cancer, individual health, and immunity strength.

In many cases, doctors don't exactly know what is happening, and since the symptoms can be similar to bacterial infections, doctors may prescribe antibiotics making the situation worse for the immune system. Absorption of nutrients get poor when good bacteria gets killed, which helps candida to proliferate even faster. Like anything else in life **cancer** is a process. It seems to develop little by little as immunity gets lower.

In order to control candida, I had to re-establish a healthy flora in my intestines with the help of probiotics, prebiotics, sauerkraut, chlorophyll-rich foods and the avoidance of commercial meats, dairy and eggs, which promote candida. Other foods that help control candida are foods that have a bitter nature. They include the sea cucumber, garlic, kelp seaweed, cerial grasses, cabbage, parsley, dandelion greens, watercress, spirullina, chlorylla and baby letttuce. I also avoided simple carbohydrates, processed foods, sweeteners and most fruits and I used only complex carbohydrates, like the sprouted millet, buckwheat, amaranth and quinoa.

Another example of how acidification affects our bodies is how it ignites **tooth decay**.

Tooth Decay and Acidification

By Dr. Sonia Warren D.D.S.

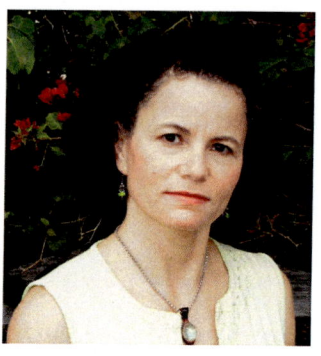

One of my first goals as a pediatric dentist is to help parents and children understand the cavity process and, with that in mind, make the changes necessary to help prevent decay. Tooth decay is caused by certain types of bacteria that live in our mouth. They attach themselves to the teeth and multiply in dental plaque. The bacteria feed on what we eat, especially obvious sugars like candy but also milk and fruit juices. There are also hidden sugars in carbohydrates (bread, potatoes, rice, pasta, etc.). Within just a few minutes of eating, or drinking sugary drinks, the bacteria begins producing acid as a by-product of its digestion of our food. Those acids lay down on the surface of the teeth and the longer we leave them there the more time they have to penetrate into the hard substance of the tooth (Enamel) and dissolve some of the minerals (calcium and phosphate). If the acid attacks are infrequent and of short duration, our saliva can help repair the damage by neutralizing the acids and supplying minerals.

However, if :

1. the mouth is dry
2. we have too many of these bacteria
3. we snack frequently; then the tooth minerals lost by attacks of acids is too great, and cannot be repaired. This is the start of tooth decay and leads to cavities. When the teeth are exposed to acids either from ingestion or from acid reflux erosion can occurre and this it evident by crater like lesions on the enamel of the teeth.

It is important to remember that the mouth is the gate for the body and having a healthy mouth and ingesting healthy foods can help maintain a balance system and health in general. The same way acids destroy the health of our teeth, acidic conditions can damage the tissues in our body.

REMOLINA DENTAL
PEDIATRIC DENTISTRY
25209 NARBONNE AVE.
LOMITA, CA 90717
310- 539-4166

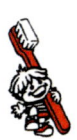

How Do You Know When You Are Out of Balance?

What are the first things you noticed in yourself? Make a point to check from time to time with yourself. Nobody, nobody, knows your body better than you. Your brain sends signals as well, check your emotional ups and downs.

A more integrative approach than Western medicine, Traditional Chinese Medicine along with Ayurveda tell us a similar story. For thousands of years, they have learned to preserve balanced health by using whole natural foods, that are pure, that come from the blue print of life, as well as managing the mind-body together to heal the whole body, as one entity in union with the universe. One common practice, mixing the five flavors of the earth; sweet, bitter, sour, pungent and salty foods in daily meals, is done to preserve a natural chemistry and a harmonious body in balanced, the preservation of yin and yang as it is known. This is where western medicine meets traditional eastern medicine. They both strike for maintaining balanced chemistry. And we know both go back to what we put in our mouth every single day. Except that eastern approaches integrate the mind- body first, putting the health of emotions and the ease of mind, that are very much linked to the health of the whole body, behind the body's physiological state.linked to the health of the whole body, before the body's physiological state.

The Many Causes of Inflammation

- Poor diet, trans fat, processed foods, excess sugar, excess salt, overeating
- Lack of exercise, stagnant energy and toxins,
- High stress and high cortisol levels
- Modified, synthetic foods
- Poor planted soils and seeds low in good bacteria and high in pesticides
- Hidden allergens such as gluten, dairy, GMOs, corn, soy
- Infections with viruses, bacteria, **yeast such as candida**, or parasites
- Toxins such as mercury, and pesticides
- Molds- mycotoxins and dangers of black mold in workplaces, homes

In many cases, inflammation is a saver, it is designed to help us survive and alert the body systems when something is not right. Without it we probably would die with so many bacteria and fungi attacks. The problem is that just as it alerts immunity and helps fight and destroy germs, it can also kill us by creating an array of distress in the body, attacking our organs from the gut lining to tissues, joints, liver, kidney, all the way to our heart. Any organ or system with constant inflammatory response is at risk of being destroyed by chronic inflammation. Like in the case of autoimmune diseases. It's even worse when we don't see it, which is usually the case, we might just feel out of balance at the beginning, and don't pay enough attention to the signs the body is sending us. Therefore, allowing inflammation to grow to the point where it becomes an extreme situation for the cells in that particular area of the body. Hence, a system gets out of balance. Avoiding extremes is key to preserveing health. This is another example how yin and yang works in the body. Extreme, chronic inflammation can kill us, but a lack of inflammatory response would not let us survive as children or when we are sick. The ideal for longevity is maintaining inflammation in balance, as it is meant to be.

Most chronic diseases such as cancer reflect a similar path: acidification, long term inflammation, and then development of the chronic disease. Cleansing our body filters: liver, lungs, kidneys by using regularly high-water content foods like vegetables and fiber foods helps maintain a slightly more alkaline blood pH, and the draining of toxins will allow more oxygen into the cells. Oxygen is nutrient number one for healthy cells. Cancer cells are anaerobic. Hence exercise, breathing techniques, chlorophyll foods and green vegetables are extremely important to keep cancer at bay. A balanced pH is crucial for preserving health and harmony in our mind-body.

chapter 3

IMMUNITY

"Nutrition is the sum total of all that we bring to the table - body, mind, heart, and soul."

— Marc David, MA

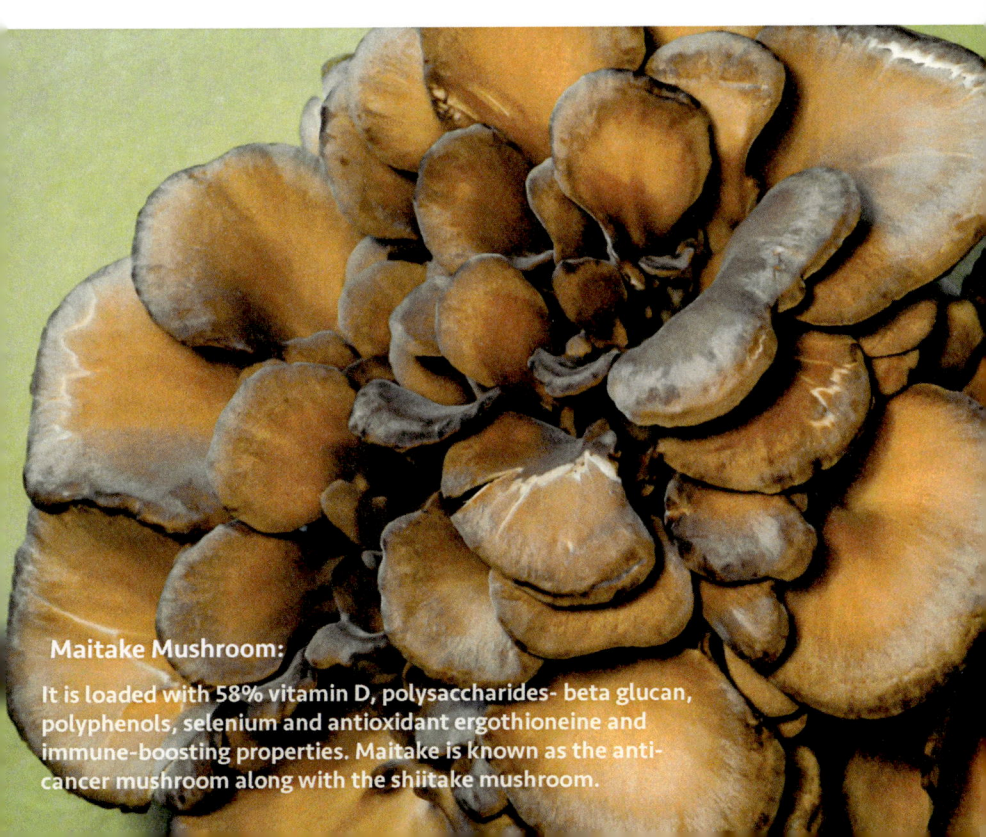

Maitake Mushroom:

It is loaded with 58% vitamin D, polysaccharides- beta glucan, polyphenols, selenium and antioxidant ergothioneine and immune-boosting properties. Maitake is known as the anti-cancer mushroom along with the shiitake mushroom.

What is the Immune System?

I really didn't understand the power of the immune system until I got sick. Cancer made me very aware of it. At the time I didn't make the connection between health and a good, normal immune system. So, I decided to learn in depth about my defense system, how it works, what lowers my defenses, and what would give power to my body's homeland security defense system. Here are some of my findings from my learning process and what it takes to maintain a happy defense system versus an overactive, constantly alert and tired one.

The immune system is a flock of cells and organs in the body working together to defend your body. It is the most complex system in the body. Its job is to defend and protect you from invaders like viruses, infections, candida, cancer, parasites, toxins that enter your body and even high levels of cortisol from stress. It is everywhere in the body, It is not localized, it doesn't work alone and it is not a single organ.

There are special immune cells that defend the body from outside or inside invaders, from the foods that we eat, the air that we breathe, the water we drink, and contact with other people as well as chemical exposures and radiation in daily life. Nowadays we have more pollutants, radiation and chemicals in our lives than what our ancestors and even our parents did when they were young. Our defense system has to adapt and work harder to protect us from every type of infection, pesticides (our conventional food supply has tone of it), toxins and of course today's high air pollution. According to a report from the world Health Organization in 2012 "Air pollution caused one in eight deaths". The majority of the deaths associated with air pollution were heart disease, stroke, chronic obstructive pulmonary disease and lung cancer.

Research has already identified at least 20 different types of immune cells and new ones are still being discovered. We hope our immune system is adapting and creating new defense cells according to our environment needs. Sometimes the immune cells adapt to new invaders. Other times it will just create allergic reactions or autoimmune responses as it seems to be the case with high pesticides in synthetic and GMO foods. These pesticides are found in our water as well. Many people, especially children, are developing high allergic reactions, a possible response of the immune system, which doesn't recognize such substances and creates anti-bodies. Hence, food allergies and inflammatory bowel syndrome are more common now than they were 20 or 30 years ago.

One of the jobs of the immune system is to defend

each organ inside of you. In order to perform its job it needs to communicate well throughout the whole body. Passing information, storing it, creating files from memories of what happened in the fights, when and how they perform against specific type of situations or invaders, so it knows what to do next time they encounter a fight. The immune cells are very well informed, since without proper communication they cannot perform very well.

The immune system's cells have a community of cells that share information throughout the body. We have more than 30 different organs and about 100 trillion cells. Many different types of cells are involved in the immunity work. Starting with the bone marrow where your red and white cells are created, then ending the process in the spleen where cells are taken off circulation when ready to die. There are specific places in the body where the immunity cells gather and share information, and use that information to gain the strength needed to perform their job.

The thymus is one of the most important places for the immune system to exchange information. Also, in the spleen where blood routes around, it is critical for immune cells to receive information on what's happening, learn how other immune cells have dealt with invaders in the past, encode all the information and store it. Here they decide what cells are getting too old to perform the job. And so from here old cells are taken out of circulation to die.

The Lymphatic System and Free Radicals

One well known area is the lymphatic system. Cancer survivors in particular know the importance of this system, for we are very much used to hearing about lymphatic fluids. Completely different from the circulatory system, the lymphatic system is in charge of circulating lymph fluids. Just as the blood runs throughout the body, the lymphatic fluids cleanse the tissues and circulate back to the heart with the movement and contraction of muscles and gravity. Therefore it is important to move and exercise. When we are active we are helping the movement of lymphatic fluids and detoxification processes. The two main jobs of the lymph fluids are to circulate nutrients and pick up the leftover waste in the tissues. There we find the lymphocytes, known as T cells and B cells, packed in the lymph nodes where they protect us from invaders, while bad cancerous cells try to go into the bloodstream to grow. When there is trouble, the nodes can be enlarged or swollen, indicating the T cells or B cells are in a battle, fighting invaders from viruses, infections or cancer cells.

At the beginning of my healing journey I thought the main indicator of good immunity was the white cell count. Doctors always checked my white cell count since it was below range and I wanted to bring them back into normal range without using drugs. So I started being more proactive, learning about white cells and what foods and practices help them. In other words, I focused my attention on nurturing them consistently. And that is what makes the difference, nurturing the immune system consistently is what works best. Sending the right message to the white cells, T cells, B cells, and the entire network of immune cells through powerful nutrition and a healthy lifestyle is probably the easiest way to make immune system happy. It was interesting to find that we have several types of white cells with specialized functions. Did you know we have white cells in each organ - the brain, the liver, the lungs, the kidneys as well as the lymphatic system? Now let's talk about free radicals.

Free radicals are molecules generated by cells in the body when exposed to toxins, viruses, germs and fungi. Free radicals contain extra oxygen to destroy invaders through oxidation. One common example of an oxidizing substance is hydrogen peroxide, which in the right form may help destroy yeast and fungi. However, there is more to the story, when free radicals scavengers are working they can attack normal cells too, this will actually cause good cells to become lousy-bad cells or centers for malignant cells to grow. This is one reason why we need to improve the intake of anti-oxidants, to protect normal cells. But wouldn't it be more effective to avoid having free radicals by **minimizing toxicity** in the first place? *How is your exposure to radiation these days? Do you drink filtered water only? Do you avoid BPA? Do you eat clean, fresh organic foods?*

The Eastern Perspective on Immunity

In Traditional Chinese Medicine, immunity, or protective QI, is considered the most vigorous and strong type of energy in the body. According to the Yellow Emperor, the oldest book in Chinese medicine teachings, the immunity energy is derived from essential substances in food and in the air that we inhale (oxygen). There is a concept in Western medicine that also indicates the importance of absorbing nutrients and utilizing oxygen for good immunity. Both Eastern and Western medicines recognized balanced immunity as the base of a good, lasting life. In his extensive research, Doctor Mark Liponis, MD, has found out that managing and paying attention to your immune system may help control the aging process, "since every disease of aging has been shown to be associated with an overactive immune system".

Most people are interested in specific foods that

promote good immunity. Yet it is not just what we eat but also the quality of the air that we breathe and how we oxygenate our lungs that has the biggest impact on the strength of our immune system. Good nutrition, movement, exercise and emotions: they all play major roles in creating happy, healthy immune cells.

The function of one area, the spleen-pancreas, is extremely important according to traditional Chinese Medicine. We are a united body in motion, with all of our body parts working together. The body organs and the mind have an effect on each other, as they are linked. Excess in work, exercise and mental activity may promote entropy (burn out) and impaired proper circulation. All of our organs work harmoniously together and self regulate. We are one body and mind. Oriental traditions see the body-mind as a whole, meaning there is a psychology associated with the organs, and there is an idea that the organs are connected to the psychology and physiology of the mind-body. In reality we are one entity and we function as such. So learning to observe the mind and the body, practicing self-care, meditation and relaxing our mind is a big part of achieving overall good health.

One example of the mind-body effect again is the spleen-pancreas. According to Oriental medicines, mental overwork can be as damaging as excess physical activity, as too many thoughts (worries) weaken the spleen-pancreas affecting its function. This causes poor nutrient absorption, and an overly alert immune system. Remember that from the Western perspective the spleen is also very important, since it acts as a route for blood/lymph circulation where immune cells gather and exchange information as well. Both Eastern and Western perspectives see the spleen-pancreas as an important player in our immunity. Actually, any activity in excess can result in the weakness of the organs, thereby affecting all of our systems.

Finding the middle path and respecting the rest and activity cycle helps counteract entropy. Discussing this subject reminds me of what several books on longevity mentioned about common practices among centenarians; they avoid excesses in life, they take breaks daily, especially when feeling tired, and they manage stressful situations with ease. Perhaps we need to learn from the happy, healthy centenarians.

Our emotions are also monitored by our immune system. According to Dr. Deepak Chopra, who mentions some of the studies in Epigenetics (outside the geno structure), "emotions can create biological responses", positive or negative. Meditation, for example, can lower high blood pressure and help control arythmias. On the other hand, fear is percieved by the immune system as a threat - a warning of a possible problem. We know that the immune system and the nervous system closely work together so that one always perceives what the other feels. They talk back and forth constantly. So thoughts, feelings and emotions influence the activity and work of our immune system. Awareness and understanding of how they work and how to nurture these areas in our body (and mind) will help the immunity cells be at ease and therefore work more effectively against cancers and other degenerative diseases.

The connection between mind-body emotions and feelings is clear. Imagine a liver overworking 24 hours, filtering the blood of a person that eats junk with poor quality oils, excess fats, and pesticides while taking medicines. That liver is overheated by the extra work it has to do on a daily basis than the liver of a person who eats more fresh, organic vegetables, eats light in general, sleeps well, and exercises regularly. In this case, toxins are circulating and getting out of the body faster, which means better blood and healthier cells. However, the first person would be more irritable and impatient and feel heavy, slow, and tired from the amount of work that the liver has to do in order to cleanse toxins. In most cases, the states of the mind reflect exactly how the organs are feeling and functioning.

Biorhythms, Patterns and Immunity

Like all of the systems in our body, our immune system works in a rhythmic flow in order to achieve balance. Everywhere, from our body to our environment, from the universe to the microbes, we can find a pattern and see that we all function in cycles and rhythms. **Everything works in rhythmic patterns.** Think of light: light is made of pulsating waves, and atoms move in pulsating waves as well. Our heart also beats in a pulsating rhythm, and our circulatory and respiratory systems are rhythms too. We have thousands of rhythms in our body that are working together, keeping the harmony of the body. Rhythms are part of our nature, so much that we even feel great with music and rhythmic movements. Equally, when some biorhythms are off, they can create chaos and miscommunications throughout the body, especially affecting immunity. Keeping the right balance within all of our systems and biorhythms is crucial to the immune system's work.

Centuries ago, ancient cultures were very observant (well.. they didn't have the TV, the internet or phones to distract them). They observed the natural rhythm of the opposites, the yin and the yang happening in our body and all of the processes in our lives. Everything in the universe has its opposite to balance it out, including our body. We are yin when we absorb in energy, which is the intake of energy into the system, from the foods that we eat to the air we breathe and water we drink. While they all provide us with the energy that comes in, Yin is always coming in. Yin is the intake of any energy or anything that we absorb. It could be information, learning something, seeing something. What you are doing right now is creating yin within, since you are taking in ideas, information. Yang, on the other hand, is the concept of expanding or letting the yin energy out. This means that we spend or give energy out while we do something, whether it's expressing, working, playing, teaching, or writing. I'm spending my energy by writing. In order to give out this energy (yang) I absorbed the energy learning (yin) and now I can expand it or let it out. I'm reutilizing the energy by giving it out, so the energy continues to move around as it should be. Energy is meant to be moving around. It is a rhythmic motion. This is why we need to preserve balance, especially when we eat, for too much energy coming in needs to be balanced by its release, reutilizing the energy.

Our immune system works in a yin and yang rhythmic pattern as well. It is balanced when we eat, exercise, and sleep properly and consistently. Rest and activity in moderation is key for good health. When we maintain rhythmic patterns in our lives, all of our processes function in a balanced flow. See the importance of giving time to our basic needs? Eating at the same time, chewing well with each bite, having time to relax, exercising regularly, sleeping at night time when we are supposed to sleep, breathing deeply in a rhythmic way and not in a stressful way. Those and other patterns will form our body's natural rhythm, which in time will create our immune and other body systems flow in a harmonious balance. Overworking immunity is like when an employee is burned out from too much work. An overactive immune system is linked to inflammation in a CRP test or C-reactive protein. I request a CRP from my doctor everytime I have a physical, and I keep records of the tests.

For many months before I got sick, I was giving too much yang: giving, giving and giving my energy out too often, overworking, not sleeping well, not resting when I felt tired, giving attention (energy) to others, not to my body's signs and needs. At the time I didn't even notice it, I just felt tired, stressed and overwhelmed.I believe that we are the center, we can preserve the balance without going on one side or the other, just like the yin and yang rhythm maintains the body in balance. Preserving my rhythmic yin and yang in balance has been one of my major goals. Are your natural biorhythms in tune? Do you feel in balance with your life and your life routines? Is your protector, your immune system, happy?

The immune system is like our homeland security, it is our protector. It doesn't work alone. It is a network of cells that are in constant communication with other systems in the body. Preserving yin-yang rhythmic balance within our natural biorhythms, avoiding extremes in diet, work, activity and lifestyle promotes a normal non-overactive immunity. Sending the right message to immune cells through powerful nutrition, positive emotions, meditation, exercise, enough rest and a healthy lifestyle is probably the easiest way to make our immune system happy, as well as minimizing toxicity from foods (pesticides), polluted water, air and toxic emotions is crucial for not overworking our best ally, the immune system.

The Five Flavors (continued from page 17):

Bitter flavor has a natural yin quality, which causes contractions and encourgaes the energy of the body to descend. Also, it dries fluids and drains dampness. Many bitter foods and herbs have a purgative effect. It is helpful for inflammations, infections and constipation. **Pungent** flavor includes acrid, spicy, hot foods and has a yang expansive property. It stimulates the circulation of energy and blood, disperses mucus, clears the lungs and improves digestion. **Sour** flavor has a yin cooling quality, causes contraction, has an astingent effect in the body and helps reverse abnormal leakage of fluids. It's more active in the liver and counteracts the effects of rich, greasy foods, helping detoxification and digestion.

chapter 4

MANAGING STRESS

"No one else can choose your attitude for you. Your perspective and choice of attitude gives you the power to be in control."

-Irene Dunlap

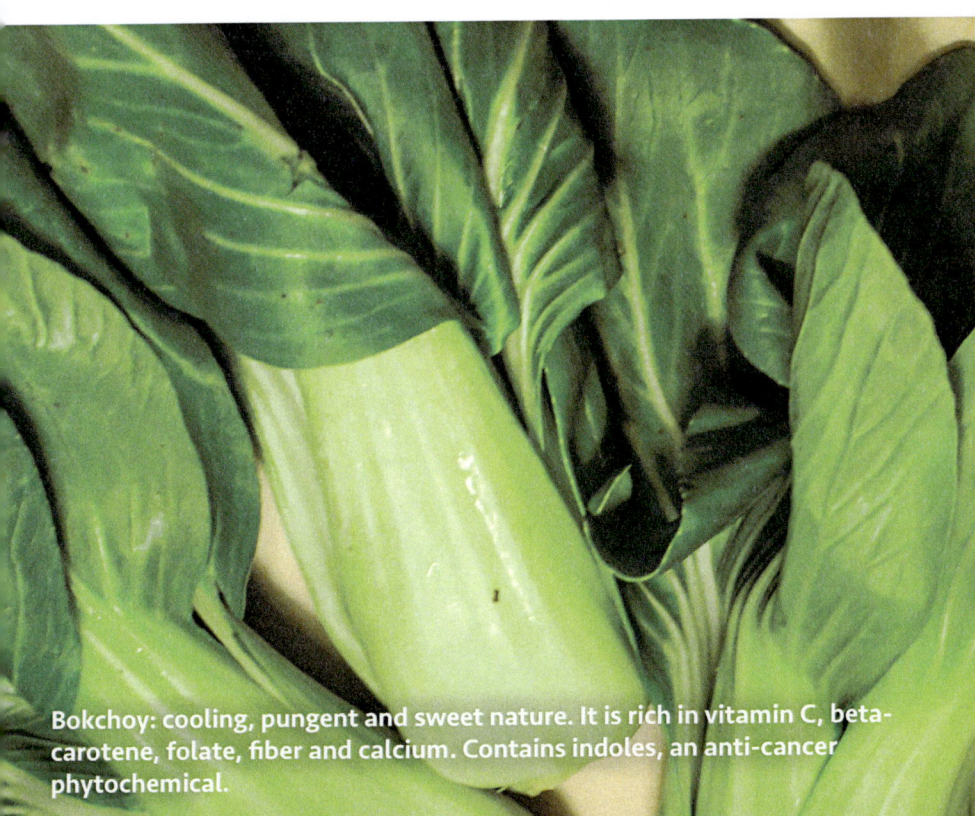

Bokchoy: cooling, pungent and sweet nature. It is rich in vitamin C, beta-carotene, folate, fiber and calcium. Contains indoles, an anti-cancer phytochemical.

High Cortisol Levels and Inflammation

A high stress level is probably one of the most common causes of the elevated hormone cortisol. High cortisol promotes and contributes to acidic blood or acidic conditions in the body, which accumulate and overtime can contribute to inflammatory diseases like cancer. Being aware of the end effects of stress has helped me, and many of my clients, create routines to maintain healthy levels of stress in our lives.

Stress is a part of life, especially in these modern times. Most of us have some kind of stress daily, so the question is: can we manage constant high stress levels to keep them from harming our health? Everybody has a different amount of stress, so we need to learn to manage our individual stressors.

For years I've certainly searched for, studied and practiced methods to control my individual stress response, I made this my goal since it is the key for good health to maintain balanced levels of cortisol. One of many sources of information that has grasped my attention is Doctor Sonia Lupien, a neuroscientist from Canada. She is an expert on stress and has been doing research on it for more than 20 years. In her studies she mentions that having small amounts of stress is actually good for the brain, as it makes us move forward and gives the brain a boost. Stress actually makes the brain more awake because there is some kind of excitement involved. It seems that stress can be helpful in certain situations when it is present in small amounts, according to Dr. Lupien. Her book, *Well Stressed: Manage Stress Before it Becomes Toxic*, has been helpful for understanding what my perception of stress is, and how to manage it in a healthy way by keeping cortisol levels in range, which helps me avoid the toxicity from acidic blood pH and promotes my immune system to be at ease at the same time.

   As with most things in life, anything in moderation is good. Even stress can be good! The problem comes around when things go to extremes, making our center, the yin and yang, out of balanced.

Chronic stress has been linked to many diseases, including cancer, diabetes, cardiovascular disease, depression, high blood pressure, high cholesterol, loss of brain function and memory problems.

How Do We Manage Stress?

Stress, like anything else, is a bio-individual response, and everybody needs to find what works for their own individual needs. We all have different needs, scientists like Lupien point out that the stress of men is totally different from the stress of women, and the stress of children. My perception on a threat has a lot to do with my unique past experiences. Also, what I eat and how I sleep will make me more vulnerable when an unexpected situation comes along. So everyone has a unique response to stressful situations depending on experiences, habits, gender, age, and of course nutrition, since the chemistry and nutrients affect the thinking process and the nervous system.

I have seen that for most people, including many of my clients, creating healthy routines to release stress results in overall good health. We know that the first step is managing the stress energy before it actually thrives or grows, not even allowing stress to the point of being unhealthy, toxic. How much stress do you feel comfortable with? Can you tell when you are experiencing beneficial stress, like the kind that occurs while planning a meaningful and interesting project, apart from harmful stress, which is more of a sense of a rush, a constant feeling of worry and dread.

The Benefits of Awareness

Many studies have shown that it is best to be aware and act before stress strikes. Awareness is the ability to be in the moment and to understand how you're feeling at a given time. Awareness connects me with my feelings, sensations and patterns. In Asian traditions awareness have been linked to remaining balanced. By being a hundred percent in the moment I'm aware of my body's signs, my mental activity and the reactions and patterns in my organs. This means I'm present in body and mind. Awareness brings me back to center, putting me into balance, which helps counteract the reaction of stress.

There are several awareness practices that contribute to my wellness and to my ability to remain centered in the middle of stressful situations. These practices include good nutrition, which helps build up my centeredness, and promotes equanimity. Breathing is most commonly known to depict our states of mind and health. Short halo breathing is linked to stress. On the other hand deep, slow and easy breathing is known to calm the mind, making us feel at ease, more centered, more balanced. Practices like meditation, yoga, tai chi have been used for thousand of years by many cultures that have adapted to changes in life, perhaps that is one reason why they are ancient cultures and still remain strong.

Breathing practices, imagery, visualization, meditation and of course the number one anti-stress tool, physical exercise, are excellent tools when practiced consistently. It doesn't need to be extraneous exercise. Actually moderate rhythmic exercise has been shown to work magnificent. Again keeping it simple works better than stressing the body, and going to extremes. Probably the easiest tool to use anywhere, anytime is breathing techniques. I use it especially at night when getting in bed if I notice my mind is still overactive. I can do this easily; in a count of four I inhale, and then I exhale on a count of eight. It is an slow release on the exhale. I do a round of 3 inhales and exhales, and by the time I finish, my breathing is more deep and relaxed and my mind is also at ease. The goal is the release of negative energy, which helps lower cortisol levels, preventing stress from thriving. The same effect happens with yoga, which is essential for channeling our chi or QI energy.

The importance of relaxation has been well-documented. Dr. Herbert Benson, at Harvard University, has shown in his research that we have the ability to reduce our heart rate, blood pressure, and brain wave activity through what he calls "the relaxation response". The response is like a mirror image of the stress response, and employs the parasympathetic system, the rest-and- response system, to reduce high stress levels. Dr. Benson found that during meditation, subjects dramatically decrease their heart rate, blood pressure and breathing rate, revealing a powerful connection between the mind and body responses.

Rhythm, Movement and Stress

Back in 2003, as I was recuperating from surgery in moments of high stress, I was looking to move slowly. I started soft yoga movements to help heal my body. It was so beautiful to see how the body and mind responded well to gentle exercises. Since I had time I decided to keep track and observed the body-mind, and the results were clear. Movement, exercise, yoga, tai chi - they all contributed to my healing and contributed to the channeling of my energy to the right direction lowering stress after the surgery and strong cancer treatments.

According to Traditional Chinese Medicine, it is wise to continue moving as much as possible (without harming the body of course), after trauma. TCM states that it is a way of promoting the **natural circulation** of fluids, **rhythms** and patterns of the body to comeback to balance, which, over time, helps the healing process. Also, modern findings have shown that when combining movement with rhythm, like in rhythmic exercise, we can enjoy a double benefit of exercise and lower the inflammation levels. It seems the body and minds enjoyment of rhythm goes beyond what we know. Good rhythm helps us turn a stressful negative energy into a positive energy for the body and state of mind, just like the sound of good rhythmic music can as well. It is all connected! What type of exercise do *you* prefer? Do you have an exercise routine? Have you noticed the difference in your stress level after practicing exercise or yoga? Make a point to notice how you feel after you exercise or do a yoga session. *Look for that feeling of ease, keep that feeling with you, breath it, store it in your brain* - those are natural states and we want to hold on to those feelings. These moments of awareness are super valuable in moments of stress. Use them, bring them back when you need them most, *don't allow moments of distress to grow*. Break down the pattern of unease as soon as you feel it coming.

Breaking the Pattern of Unease

Nowadays, looking at my clients lives and stresses, I see that most people do better when they have healthy outlets to release negative stress, but what really caught my attention are those people who can control stress before it strikes, even when they are busy professionals with tight schedules.

The one common denominator between these people is that they eat mostly a plant-based diet, high in leafy greens, whole grains, beans and organic produce, which provides them with good amounts of minerals; like calcium, magnesium, manganese and zinc making them more calm and able to handle the stressors better. Whole nutrition, free of processed sugars, white flours, synthetic foods, additives and chemicals makes a huge difference in handling stress. Whole nutrition creates a smooth and even energy in the mind, versus poor empty nutrition from processes foods, chemicals and high sugars, which creates uneven energy resulting in unease thinking. As stated in TCM and Ayurveda, Whole nutrition makes us complete, even when things are stressful. Whole nutrition keep us rooted, centered without tilting toward extremes. Whole nutrition help our body's yin and yang stay in rhythmic balance even in the middle of changes.

I have a habit of questioning the energy of the foods, epecially when I'm in a restaurant or eating out, I remind myself of eating the right foods as I'm checking the menu with the question in my mind: what type of ENERGY is in this food? Because I know that whatever I put IN me will reflect OUT in the energy I will have in a few hours after the meal or even in the next days. This habit reminds me to put good whole energy within my own body consistently, instead of empty caloric energy that wont help my body be healthy and wont help my mind handle stressors calmly.

I have a written note that I go to when stressful times or situations are coming. It is a reminder of the foods and practices that keep me in balance. Yoga, dancing and meditation, these are some of the resources I use the most, along with walking my dog and getting out of the house to do deep breathing. Gardening is one of my favorites, as being in touch with nature helps release negative energies. When I am feeling out of balance or I see possible stressful situations are coming , then I keep looking at my note, I don't ignore it; I actually observe myself, and look at my note. It's a reminder of what I do when I feel stress is trying to grow. It seems the key is to preserve that center and ease even when chaos is around us. What would *your* list look like? What things do *you* know help *you* keep balance in your life? What type of foods would *you* crowd out and which would you reach out to?

Signs and Symptoms of High Stress:

- Fatigue
- Sleep disorders
- Anger
- Inability to concentrate
- Muscle tension
- Tight neck and shoulders
- Tightness in chest
- Reduced sexual drive
- Constipation and/or diarrhea
- Hair loss
- Nervousness and/or anxiety
- Sadness and/or depression
- Moodiness

We all have stressors in our lives. Finding our balance, especially in times of chaos and tension is crucial for avoiding acidic blood pH from high cortisol, which is the result of constant stress, and when our nervous systems and mind are in high alert or overly active. Calming the brain and the stress response before it fully develops help us bring cortisol levels down. Being aware of your thoughts, and feelings helps you detect stress before it becomes unhealthy. Awareness is your early warning system. Especially when you connect with your natural rhythmic breathing, which will send signals to other systems and biorhythms helping the whole body and mind find that place of ease. Creating the habit of being at **ease** *more often will help the body avoid* **disease***. Regular meditation is one easy habit for calming down tension before it becomes stress. More than other diseases, cancer, has been directly linked to high stress levels.*

chapter 5

DIGESTION AND CANCER

"To keep the body in good health is a duty, otherwise we shall not be able to keep our mind strong and clear."

-Budha

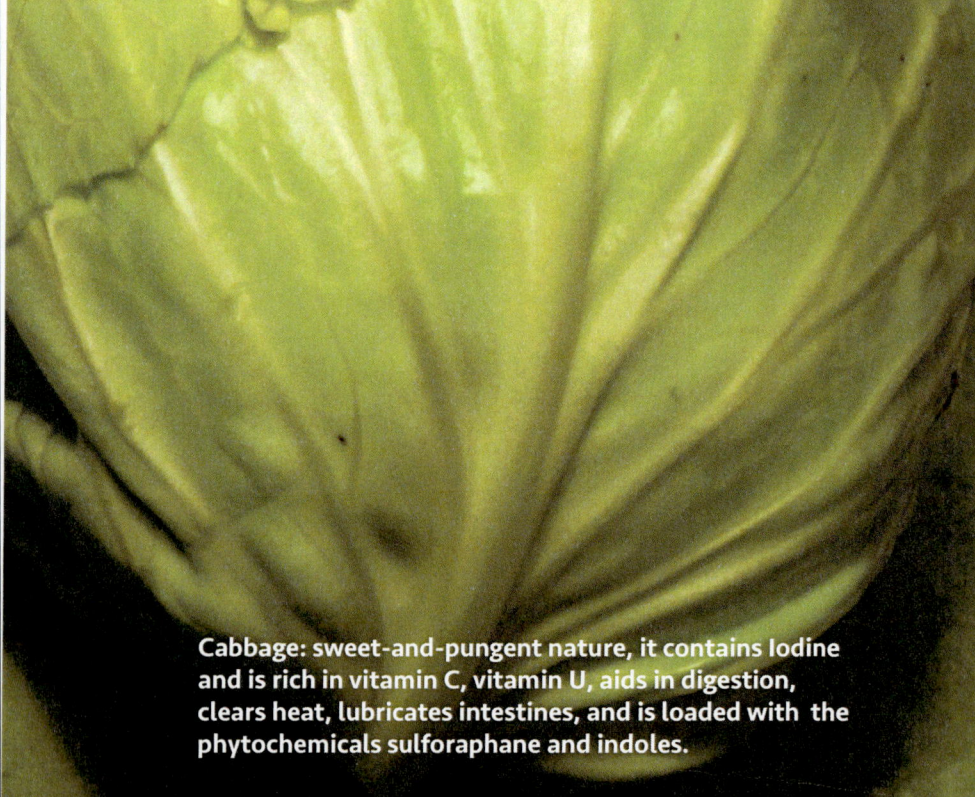

Cabbage: sweet-and-pungent nature, it contains Iodine and is rich in vitamin C, vitamin U, aids in digestion, clears heat, lubricates intestines, and is loaded with the phytochemicals sulforaphane and indoles.

D igestion is the process of breaking food down into components that are small enough to be absorbed by the body. Digestion happens before the entry of nutrients into the circulation. Absorption is the movement of nutrients, including water, across the intestinal wall and into blood or lymph.

The Digestive System includes the mouth, esophagus, stomach, pancreas, liver, gallbladder, and small/large intestines. *The Digestive system does not work alone, as other systems participate in the process. Here are the other systems and processes involved:*

- •Endocrine system: secretes hormones
- •Nervous system: sends signals that control passage of food, controls hunger
- •Cardiovascular system: transports nutrients to cells
- •Urinary system and Integumentary system: eliminate waste

Looking at nutrition as the root of energy, we see the importance of having a healthy gastrointestinal system (G.I.) and its ability to extract nutrients from our gut. The GI is a long hollow tube of about 30 feet in length. The GI is our center, our digestive trunk. Yes! We have a trunk, just like trees have a trunk, it holds our roots (the intestines) and keeps the whole body unified, stable and nourished. The transit time within the GI is affected by the composition of the diet, food preparation, physical activity, emotions, temperature, medications, and illnesses.

Our center, as it is called in Traditional Chinese Medicine (TCM), is our digestive tract; it keeps all of our body parts unified and it is responsible for feeding the whole body. We have two arms, two legs, two lungs, two kidneys, and one long G.I. It is our center. Its job is extremely important. It is in charge of providing us with usable nutrients, processing and transforming nutrients into energy, and also getting rid of waste on a daily basis. It is good to remember that we eat to obtain energy, that food is fuel, but food has to be transformed and absorbed first in order to become the fuel for life. Eating doesn't imply good nutrition. What's most relevant is absorbing the nutrients properly. We need a healthy Digestive system to process foods and get the **fuel** for life, **energy**.

Digestion starts in the mouth. TCM and other holistic practices believe that a person can survive and fight diseases as long as their digestive tract is functioning well. In fact, five thousand years ago, Chinese physicians declared "Health begins at the mouth". Healing our digestive tract from mouth to colon is a major factor in recovery from and avoidance of illnesses, especially chronic diseases like diabetes, arthritis, cancer, lupus, heart conditions and brain issues as well, which you will learn more about in the next pages.

Why Does Digestion Influence Our Immune System?

An astonishing 70% of the immune system is located in or around the digestive tract. Our immunity is constantly protecting our GI from invaders and from foods that contain pesticides and bacteria, from spoiled foods, from non-recognizable components like chemicals, foreign elements and even from synthetic foods that might be unrecognizable. One common case we see nowadays is the link between genetically modified foods (GMOs), and gastrointestinal problems. It seems the pesticides in the seeds of GMOs, especially the component glyphosate, are causing the immune system to react by creating constant allergic reactions and inflammations. This is probably why we see more allergies nowadays than we did twenty years ago. However, the pesticides that keep our immune system overly alert are not the only problem. According to many sources, articles, and even health documentaries, doctors and scientists agree on one thing: pesticides in GMOs and conventional foods also affect the capacity of absorption from our gut. Mainly because these pesticides act just like antibiotics do in our gut, by killing the bad and the good bacteria. This bacteria influences the bio-diversity of microbes in the soil. And at the same time it affects the micro bio-diversity in our gastrointestinal tract. So our gut and the soil are in constant communication, which affects our absorbtion of nutrients. Remember, we are connected to nature at a deep level, especially through the communication between microbes. The microbes have a purpose in the circle of life. I was astonished to see the similarity between microbes in the soil and the microbes in our GI at a conference with Dr. Miller, one of the experts on this topic. These microbes look alike and they serve the same purpose at a different level. The microbes in the soil contribute to the absorption of nutrients, especially minerals for the plants to be healthy and strong. The micro bio-diversity in our gut contributes to our wellness, energy, and our ability to absorb and process nutrients. The more micro-diversity we have, the better we can expect our bodies to function, and the reverse is true, less micro-diversity in our gut means less nutrients, less energy for our body and probably more cravings and hunger.

One way pesticides, like glyphosate, kill weeds is by not allowing the roots to soak up the nutrients from the soil. This weakens the plants, lowers their nutritional and mineral content, and eventually causes them to die. When we ingest pesticides, our gut reacts in the same way, on a smaller scale at the beginning, then the reaction accumulates. We receive less and less nutrients from the foods that we eat. Our gut doesn't extract nutrients in its full capacity. At the same time the immune system is spending lots of our energy fighting the non-recognizable DNA from GMOs and pesticides, and this creates an inflammatory response that comes from the reactions of antibodies. Immunity deals with lots of pesticides and pollution as it is constantly assessing what's good and normal and what's bad. Remember, 70% of your whole immune system is located around the G.I. It has been trained to manage and deal with invaders for thousands of years, but in these last decades new inventions in pesticides and modified foods have created organisms that never existed in the world before affecting the DNA of foods, so it confuses our immune system which cannot recognize them, and it reacts against them as it would against new invaders.

One way we can help our immune and digestive systems is by eating organic foods, which posses a normal DNA and have been shown to provide more nutrients. The organic plants are healthier, they provide more minerals and vitamins to our bodies, and they are free of pesticides. With organic foods, the immune system has less work to do and can really focus on defending us from major diseases instead of being overwhelmed with constant alerts from allergic reactions. As I was writing this section, I remembered that years ago, as I was going through chemo, my body reacted really well when I switched to eating organic foods only. I guess I helped my gut extremely, as organic foods gave me back the micro-diversity I needed it at the time to absorb the nutrients that helped replenish my health after the treatments. (Cancer treatments may also affect the lining of the G.I., especially when the intestines like in my case got affected by radiation). So the renewal of the G.I. gets easier as we provide the right micro-diversity through organic, wholesome vegetables and produce, especially leafy greens.

The health and chemistry of the soil where food

is planted matters too! The chemistry of the soil needs to be balanced, and ecologically organic in order to provide us with the nutrients and the organisms that we need in order to have a normal, healthy GI and thereby have a happy, healthy mind-body.

Specialist in gut health Dr. Irina Matveikova explains the importance of microflora balance in the avoidance of abnormal formations in the colon: "Microflora in the digestive tract play an important role in the proliferation and differentiation of the intestinal epithelium. The bacteria that live in close proximity to the cells of our intestines help control the growth and reproduction of the epithelial cells. They help control genetic expression in the intestines, insuring that they are functioning normally. Intestinal cells are exposed to proteolytic bacteria (putrefactive microbes, such as clostridia, that are a normal part of gut flora and secrete toxins such as ammonia). These bacteria can proliferate in an uncontrolled manner, causing the formation of polyps (in some cases, precancerous lesions) in the colon walls, which; these polyps if not excised in time, may lead to colon cancer."

"Balanced intestinal microflora are essential

for the development and maturation of a normal immune system, both systemically (for the general defense of the body against external infections) and locally (through the intestinal mucosa). Distributed throughout the digestive tract are various types of immunocompetent cells (immune cells, such as T-cells, that function normally following exposure to an antigen) and lymphoid follicles, similar to the tonsils, that are associated with the digestive system. The good bacteria train the immune system to defend itself; they help it form and maintain immunological memory, competing with pathological and harmful bacteria for food and space. They also nourish our mucosa. The balance of this system can be upset after a course of antibiotics or other medications, as a result of chronically elevated stress levels, or due to an unhealthy diet. This imbalance may show up as frequent infections, digestive problems, and general health disorders."

Unfortunately we see more and more G.I. problems in our society nowadays, probably due to a diet that lacks foods with natural fiber, such as beans, whole grains, vegetables, and fruits. The use of low quality oils and chemically treated, genetically modified foods seems to also contribute to these issues.

Common digestive problems include: Acid Reflux, IBS, IBD (Crohn's or Ulcerative Colitis), Lactose Intolerance, Constipation/Diarrhea, Celiac Sprue, Gallstones, Diverticulitis

Eat Light, Live Longer

You can digest enzymatically—feel good, have clearer thinking and more energy. Or you can digest fermentively—feel sluggish, tired, bloated, and have unclear cloudy thinking.

"Eat Light, Live Longer!" is an old Asian saying. Ancient cultures like the Chinese, the Hindu, and the Japanese put an emphasis on one thing: in order to survive and stay healthy we need to have, first and foremost, good digestion. It makes sense, as we know digestion influences our immune system. Overeating, for example, plays a huge toll in overworking immune cells in the gut. At the same time, overeating, instead of producing more energy, takes away the energy we already have. This leaves us feeling tired, since our immune system goes into a battle with the bacteria fermenting the food that didn't get digested. Bad bacteria is happy when we overeat, and it feeds and proliferates from the non-digested extra food. This battle between our immunity and the bacteria creates a lot of of work for our defense system, as it becomes increasingly alert when the leftover food is not broken down completely due to the lack of enzymes. We can put only so much food into our stomach. The amount of food depends on the size of the stomach, the enzymes that the pancreas produced and, of course, the hydrochloric acid and the digestive messages.

Eating Only When We're Hungry

This is another common great habit of centenarians. They eat only when they are hungry and they don't let emotions or society control their eating habits. Eating at the moment of hunger contributes to the regulation of insulin, the response of hormones and most importantly, the effective absorption of nutrients. So we don't waist time, money and energy, we actually gain more energy when eating only when we are hungry. It sets the GI into a routine so it sends signals and messages when to eat, and when to stop eating. In general it helps us maintain our natural rhythms, a healthier GI and a healthier immune system as well.

Doing a hunger check every day has helped me to establish the habit of eating only when I'm hungry. You can do it too! Before you put food, any food into your mouth, pause …. ask yourself "am I truly hungry?" If the answer is yes, eat and enjoy the food. If the answer is no, don't eat it. Instead take a deep breath and drink ½ glass of water or tea. Getting into this discipline has helped me to observe my behavior, analyze it and recognize when it is emotional eating, or mere social eating (doing what others are doing). It also set the stage for new habits to take place. Nowadays I can easily place my hand on my stomach and ask the question am I truly hungry? The answer is clear, my body is talking back, and I can distinguish when I am hungry. It is good to be hungry. It means my enzymes are ready to be used, just like when we break the fast at breakfast time when we are hungry, ready to eat. I like that feeling and appreciate having the foods available when I am hungry. It is a blessing to have nutritious foods when we are hungry. I would rather have small amounts of the right nutritious food than an excess of the wrong foods, which damage our body's health little by little.

Digestive Fire and Digestive Intelligence

From a holistic perspective, we are part of the environment, and the environment has an impact on our health and nutrition. The weather outside places an important role on our body's capacity to digest and absorb nutrients. Our GI works better when there is heat present. Usually on windy days and cold days we look for warm foods, since it is only natural to help the body and the digestive system to stay warm. Eating cold foods in cold weather can create dampness, which involves extra humidity, and promotes an environment in which bacteria can thrive. Digestion, just like the body, requires a specific warm temperature. Sometimes drinking cold beverages, or staying in damp places, can bring the GI into coldness or dampness, creating contractions and slowing down digestion. In order to digest well, foods need to be broken down, and in order to break down foods we need to have enough energy in the digestive organs, or what's called the "digestive fire." This is primordial for good nutrition to take place. The digestive fire is also called the "Center Burner" for a reason, since, just like a burner, it needs heat to function well. It is like your own personal heat (stove) where nutrients get broken down and extracted. Traditional Asian medicine stipulates that without a strong "Digestive Fire" and balanced gut flora, we might not be able to absorb nutrients well, even when eating nutritious, raw foods (which are cooling).

Perhaps that's why holistic nutrition suggests eating and cooking according to the seasons, to counteract the strong changes in temperatures and allow the digestive system to adapt to extreme temperature changes. Also, as we age, temperatures and energy can drop down, requiring us to prepare and eat warmer foods, soups, stews, purees and, in general, easier to digest meals. When feeding convalescent patients, many hospitals in China's rural areas prepare what's called congee, an easy to digest rice or millet soup. It is cooked for hours at low temperatures. The purpose is to give the patient a broken down nutrient-rich warm soup, which helps assimilate nutrients quickly. An easily digestible meal like this helps patients preserve their own energy during the digestive process.

I was curious to learn more about this topic as I was healing my digestion using holistic modalities. In Japanese traditions they also emphasize the importance of keeping the stomach warm, preserving the pancreatic and digestive fire. Some traditions actually suggest covering the stomach as we sleep to preserve the "candle light", as they call it. They advise against allowing wind and cold to penetrate the stomach area. Keeping the stomach area warm and protected is believed to have important health benefits.

I usually chop parsley (which is warming) to serve on top of my beans, even when the beans have been cooked with garlic, onions, and warming spices like turmeric and cayenne. Most cultures use daily warming spices when cooking, the purpose is to help the digestive process by warming up our digestive fire. I also noticed the nature's way: my dog's routine, and I have seen this in other animals as well. Most animals curl up and rest after they eat. It seems that they curl up to keep their tummy warm, and it is very natural for them to do this routine. They are probably saving energy for better digestion and to ensure the proper absorption of nutrients as they relax and warm up their digestive fire. Nature knows the way!

Doesn't it feel good when we put a hot bottle on the tummy area? I have used it before and it does create a nourishing feeling. I guess ancient traditions knew it a long time ago. The abdomen is a place of nourishment, where energy and warmth emerge from and spread throughout the whole body, and it's also a place of natural intelligence, for it communicates with the whole body-mind in more than one way.

After all our GI possesses a digestive intelligence as explained by GI specialist, Dr. Irina Matveikova in her article "Digestive Intelligence". She states that "The digestive system has tremendous neurological and hormonal potential. This is why scientists and the pharmaceutical industry are currently devoting so much research and testing to **neurogastroenterology**." The findings show several similarities between the brain and the gut. They even found the same neurons in both places. They called it the gut-brain or "second brain". These two brains are in constant communication. "The second brain neuronal function is very similar to that of the head-brain. It has an extensive network of neurons located between the two muscular layers of the digestive system walls, it has an identical structure as the neurons in the brain, and both produce similar chemical molecules—neurotransmitters and hormones necessary for proper functioning of the body". No wonder we can not even think clear when we have digestive issues, especially after cancer treatments. The famous chemo brain makes more sense now, for our head-brain is probably not able to communicate well or receive messages from the second brain, our gut-brain, when the natural flora in our gut is out of balance or when we are treated with heavy antibiotics or medications that have an adverse effect on our gut's micro-biome.

The GI has a huge impact on our emotions. Did you know that most of your serotonin, and neurotransmitters is produced in your GI? It means that the health of your GI affects your sleep, your thinking processes as well as your immune system! So what can we eat and do to promote balanced GI health?

Holistic Health, Digestion and Habits

I've been adding several natural healers and helpers to my diet in order to maintain balanced GI health. Regarding food, probably the number one vegetable to heal the gut is cabbage. Full of sulfur, vitamin U and **anti-inflammatory** and **anti-cancer** compounds, **cabbage** is well known in holistic nutrition for its healing properties. I remember years ago, as I finished cancer treatments, I started bleeding from the bladder,

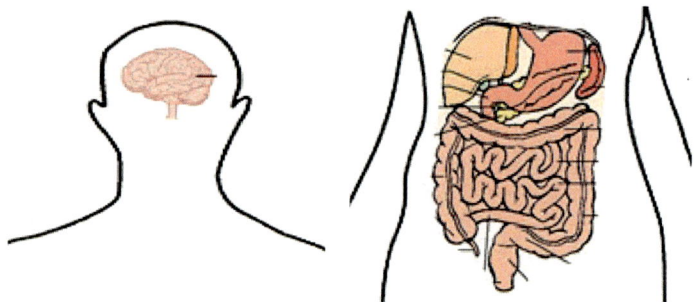

so much that doctors suggested a bladder surgery.
I was so afraid of going to the bathroom because
of the frequent bleeding. I was puzzled by the
bleeding. They called it "collateral damage" from
the radiation treatments. Since I didn't want
to have surgery, I started my search of holistic
natural ways to heal the ulcers in my bladder. I
used cabbage. It took me three months of drinking
cabbage juice every morning, consistently, until,
little by little, the bleeding stopped, and when I
went back to have the test, the bladder specialist
was puzzled to see a healed bladder after seeing
large ulcers all around it only a few months ago.
It was the natural whole compounds working
together every day, helping the delicate tissue of
the bladder to heal. I love cabbage! It is my best
friend! Not only did it help me with my bladder,
but it has also renewed and healed my gut. And
in the form of sauerkraut, cabbage is a superstar,
probably one of the best fermented foods to help
heal many GI issues. Nutrient absorption can
be poor when the gut is not functioning well. I
definitely noticed the difference in energy after
using sauerkraut for a long time. It is now an easy
habit in my eating routine. I use it as a part of my
dressings.

I also use **probiotics** and **prebiotics**. The word pro-biotic means pro life, and we know that probiotics help the gut, but not everybody knows that probiotics may not arrive alive to their destiny because the hydrochloric acid in the stomach kills them. There are many kinds of probiotics, and it is best to choose them according to GI needs, age, gender, strain diversity, and delay delivery. They should preferably be made from organic whole foods. Probiotics are actually found in foods. They feed our good bacteria, they are the fertilizers for productive bacterial growth and are made out of fructooligosaccharides (FOS) and inulin, natural sugars found in certain carbohydrates, but especially in whole grains, and other foods like burdock root, onions, chicory root, bananas, garlic, endives, dandelion root and dandelion greens, and radicchio, which happens to be one of the most studied foods for its anti-cancer properties. I definitely use them all in my recipes!

- Movement, rhythm, core training exercises and yoga have been used to strengthen digestive organs and muscles, making it easy to absorb the nutrients, helping the body's detoxification process and of course, exercise is, as we know, good for our brains, both our head-brain and our gut-brain! Which one would work for you? Which could you turn into a habit?

Serving size is crucial for maintaining good digestion.

- When serving food, I prefer small plates instead of big plates like I used to.Using smaller plates has helped me manage portion control, which helps utilize the amounts of enzymes that break down the foods that I have eaten in a meal. Therefore I can have a better absorption of nutrients and energy! This habit is key for nutrition and at the same time it helps the immune system to be at ease, which is the opposite of overeating, since overeating puts Immunity into alertness. Other great motivations to make this a habit are the clear thinking that comes with light eating, and the clear mind, better memory and feeling of ease. It is all connected!

Eating to Preserve Balance

For a moment, picture the earth from far away, as if you are looking at the earth from the moon. What do you see the most in our planet? Water. The earth is 80 to 85% water. If we look inside your body, what is your body composed mainly of? Water. Wouldn't it make sense for your plate to contain foods that are composed of mainly water?

Our plates, when we serve food, should be in sync with our environment and the way we are made, out of water, to promote that harmony it makes sense to have our plate be at least 70% composed of foods that contain water, like vegetables, and serve smaller amounts of solids like proteins. Fruits also contain large amounts of water, but they are better consumed separate.

Food Combining

After learning about the importance of digestion and absorption, many clients ask me: what are the best food combinations for easy proper digestion? Good dietary practices form an important foundation for healing, making all medicine more effective. From the holistic nutrition perspective we know that too much elaborate food encourages our taste buds to overindulge. The consequences are digestive fermentation, feelings of fatigue, contaminated

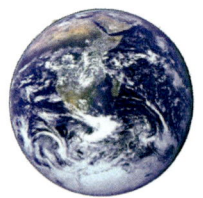 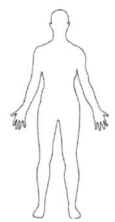 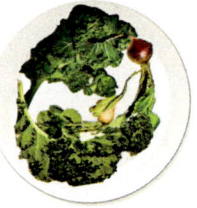

Our Earth, Our Body, Our Plate

blood, and a confused mind.

While poor food combining decreases nutrient assimilation, it can, in many cases, produce intestinal gas, abdominal pain and swelling. This is especially true when such eating practices become a habit, since, over time, they may contribute to inflammatory diseases and degenerative conditions.

Remember that proper, complete assimilation of food is a result of the action of **proper chewing** (properly liquifying foods before swallowing) and **digestive enzymes**. Different types of food, even foods within the same group, such as two different grains or seeds require their own unique enzymes. When many different ingredients are eaten at the same meal, the body becomes overwhelmed, confused and may not be able to produce all of the necessary enzymes at the right time. Hence, the digestion will take place through bacterial action, which causes yeast fermentation and putrefaction of foods in the GI. Digestive fermentation is not to be confused with the healthful, controlled fermentations such as those used in sauerkraut, miso or tempeh.

When it comes to digestion, simpler and fresher is better. Too many ingredients in a meal results in less nutrition, less energy, and digestive and mental discomfort. Eat fruit by itself and milk by itself. Try eating proteins and starches at separate meals.

Combine your proteins efficiently! Proteins are the slowest to digest and require more enzymes. Examples of effective combinations of proteins: Beans, tofu, fish, and hempcombined with non-starchy vegetables, like all leafy greens, celery, mushrooms, cabbage, broccoli, tomoatoes, and peppers. Whole grains, like quinoa, millet, brown rice, and buckwheat contain both protein and starch and they are not digested easily when combined with beans or animal proteins in the same meal, especially if you have a sensitive digestive system. They are digested easier when combined with non-starchy vegetables.

Traditional Holisitic Eating Tips ·

- Eat according to your health and constitutional needs, since everyone is unique and has different needs. Nurture your uniqueness.

- Liquids and food should not be too hot or too cold. This is especially true for people with sensitive stomachs or after having surgery or treatments. Too much heat debilitates the stomach and creates acidity, while too much coolness creates contractions of the stomach and GI organs.

- Do not be so rigid about your diet as to create a feeling of stress around food. Stress can be more poisonous than having a treat once in while.

- Relax and get comfortable, it is time to welcome your new energy through food! Relaxation helps you digest your food and sleep well at night, and by doing so you are helping your immune system in functioning. Allow a time for meals in a clean environment, surrounded with pleasant sounds, aromas, colors, and conversation. Avoid emotionally charged subjects, confused scattered talk or thoughts. Avoid eating while worried, angry, watching TV, using the computer, using the phone, reading, or before bathing.

- Drinking with meals dilutes the digestive juices. However, a small amount of warm water is ok for most people. In general, drink water or herbal teas fifteen to twenty minutes before meals, and two hours after a meal rich in carbs, proteins like grains-beans and animal proteins.

• Promoting healthy-eating routines: We are naturally set by rhythms and habitual patterns. Eating and digesting is a rhythm too, our digestive juices are produced according to the body's routines, not by our working or social schedule. The night and early morning hours before five a.m. are passive times when digestive organs need to rest. The liver in particular needs to complete many metabolic functions, which depend on the early stages of digestive activity. It especially needs to complete its task of blood purification, which is interrupted and altered when meals are eaten late in the day.

• Simple meals, or one pot meals, take little time to prepare and are easier to digest

We want to remember that an astonishing 70% of our immune system is located in or around our digestive tract, protecting our center. Our digestive system is the center where our energy start circulating. In summary, when buying ingredients, preparing meals or eating out, you can make counsious decisions and eat with a purpose in mind. If you want to be healthy, be able to avoid and fight diseases and have good energy, you want to eat to improve digestion.

LILLY'S **RECIPES**

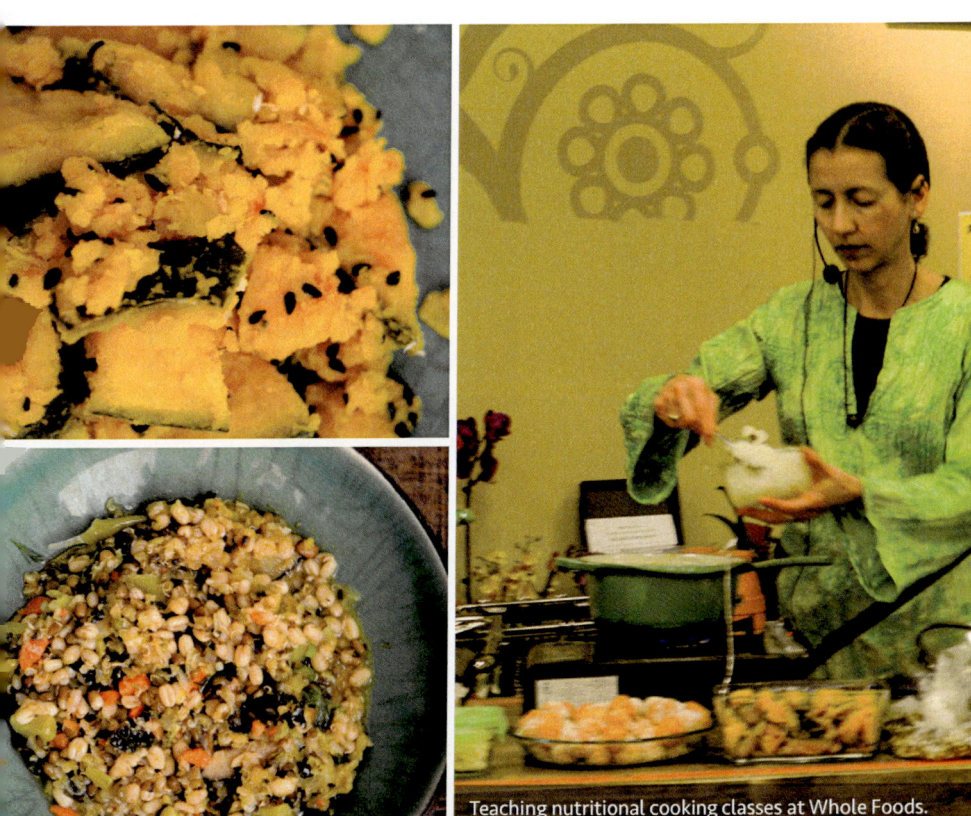

Teaching nutritional cooking classes at Whole Foods.

Lilly's Cream of Teff

Teff is a nutritional powerhouse, well known for providing stamina to Ethiopian runners. It is the smallest grain in the world, which makes it easy to digest. Contains good protein, minerals, smart carbs and good fiber .

Ingredients

¼ c. Teff grain

3 tbs. almond meal powder (grind almonds or hemp seeds)

3 tbs. oats bran

2 1/4 c. water

1/8 c. almond milk (optinal)

1 ½ teaspoon liquid vanilla , a pinch sea salt

¼ tsp. cinnamon- ¼ tsp. nutmeg powder, a pinch of cardamom powder

Fruit for sweetness (organic apple or berries)

Preparation

Put teff in water to boil, cover, boil for 8-10 minutes, stir well several times. Then add flours, fruits, spices, mix all the ingredients well. Put on low heat to cook for 5 minutes stirring several times, cover, let it cook, water should be absorbed, grains should be sticky. Check for the desired thickness, I like it thick and creamy. Add almond milk, mix it, cook for 2 more minutes, turn off. Let it stand covered for 3 minutes, serve and enjoy it! Makes 2 servings.

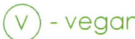 (V) - vegan

(GF) - gluten free

Lilly's Alkaline Vegetable Drink

It has wonderful alkalizing properties, great absorption of nutrients, and it is easy to do! I like to start the day with this drink as it gives me lots of energy and anti-oxidants.

Ingredients

1 c. warm water or green tea water

1 stalk organic celery, chopped

1 cup chopped organic green cabbage

1 hand full parsley leaves or ½ c.

1 hand full watercress leaves- no stems

1tbs. flaxseeds or chia seeds

½ to 1 lemon juice

1-2 tsp. bee pollen granules

3 tbs. hemp seeds

Preparation and Benefits

Blend all ingredients untill the whole juice is smooth. The fiber is great for cleansing, weight control and elimination of toxins. Warm vegetable drinks help preserve our G.I. energy and facilitate absorption of nutrients. Chia and flax seeds provide omega 3s, fiber, calcium and protein. Cabbage provides anti-cancer benefits, excellent for weigh control and beautiful skin. Watercress protects the lungs, it is pungent. This means that it helps in cleansing the liver, kidneys and lungs. Celery helps eliminate toxins, and reduce cravings and appetite. Bee pollen is a low glycemic, and offers many health benefits, like minerals and vitamins and provides great protein amino acids. Hemp seeds provide also protein and fatty acids.

Lilly's Cruciferous Green Soup

In this soup I'm combining the wonderful health and anti-inflammatory benefits of cruciferous vegetables, ginger and the Allium vegetable family of onions, garlic, green onions along with the immune boosting effects from maitake-shiitake mushrooms.

Ingredients

½ bunch kale

1 carrot medium size

1-2 stalk celery

1 ½ cup packed dandelion greens

1 ½ cup or 3 leaves green cabbage

1-2 baby bok choy

¾ cup sprouted mung beans or sprouted lentils

1 1/2 c. cilantro leaves

1/2 c. parsley leaves

7" seaweed kelp cut into tiny pieces ¼ inch (use scissors)

1 big yellow onion

 2-3 medium cloves garlic

½ tsp.teaspoon dried thyme

Sea Salt to taste

½ tsp. turmeric powder

1 tsp. fresh ginger

Cayenne pepper to taste (optional)

10 cups water or more depends how you prefer your soups

½ cup tiny-chopped green onions (to serve on top)

2 spoons olive oil (only add at the end)

1 tbs. capers

Preparation

1. In a large stockpot of medium heat put 8 cups water to boil, add 1 minced garlic clove, seaweed kelp, sprouted beans, and ½ onion chopped. Let it boil for 30 minutes. This is the broth for your soup.

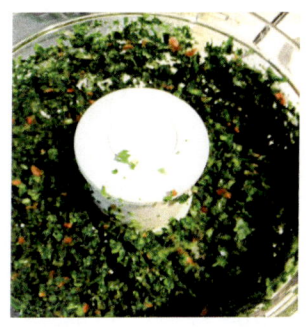

2. In a food processor, or blender, chop all greens, ginger, 1 garlic cloves, ½ onion, except 1 cup of cilantro until they are tiny (rice size like or totally blended) . Keep 1 cup to add at the end. Add the blended chopped mix of vegetables to the pot with the broth, mixing well, add salt and cayenne pepper to taste, let it boil for about 15 minutes, with lid on, then add olive oil mixing well to blend flavors, add more fresh cilantro leaves on top. Let it stand cover for 5 minutes. Serve it with pieces of avocado, cilantro, capers and green onions on top! *Enjoy the nutritious, anti-cancer properties of this cruciferous soup!*

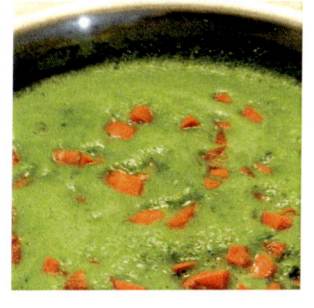

Lilly's One Pot Sprouted Meal

Sprouts and sprouted beans and grains are well-known for providing us with easy to digest proteins amino acids, great energy, fiber, vitamins and minerals!

Ingredients

1 c. sprouted mung beans or sprouted lentils
½ c. sprouted quinoa
10-11 c. spring filter water
½ cup hemp tofu
1 bag maitake or 4 shiitake mushrooms, sliced
1 large organic yellow onion, chopped
2 cloves garlic, pressed
2 c. green cabbage, chopped
1 c. broccoli, chopped
1-2 organic celery stalks, chopped
1 c. kale, chopped
5" seaweed kelp, chopped tiny pieces

Spices:
1-2 tbs. grind fresh ginger
¼ to ½ tsp. cayenne pepper
½ tsp. turmeric powder
1tsp. coriander powder
Salt to taste
½ c. chopped green onions
½ c. cilantro or parsley

Preparation

In a large stockpot of medium heat put 10 cups water to boil, add garlic, onion, seaweed, sprouted beans, quinoa, let it cook cover for 10 minutes. Then add mushrooms, hemp tofu, ginger and all chopped vegetables, cook for 15 minutes. Add water as needed.

Mix all powdered spices plus salt in one container add spices to the meal, mix well, let it cook for 5 minutes. Turn off. Let it stand for 5 minutes. Serve with fresh parsley or cilantro on top and green onions! This meal goes well with pieces of avocado on the side. *Enjoy it!*

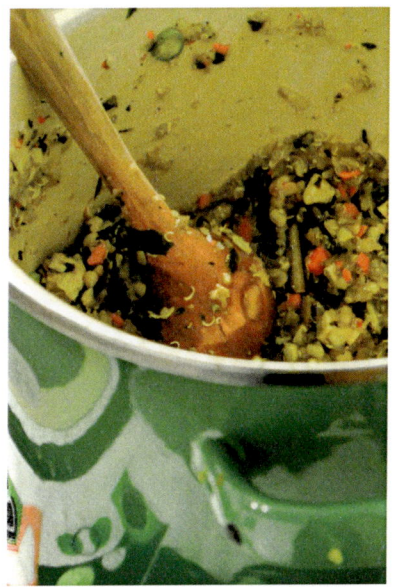

Liver Lovers-Beet Salad

The ingredients in this recipe help cleanse the liver and detoxify the blood when used frequently over a period of time.

Ingredients

2 cups cooked red beets

1/2 organic lemon zested

juice of 1 big organic lemon

1 tbs. olive oil

¼ c. cooked and chopped wakame-seaweed

pinch sea salt

1 c. chopped fresh organic parsley

1 c. dandelion greens chopped

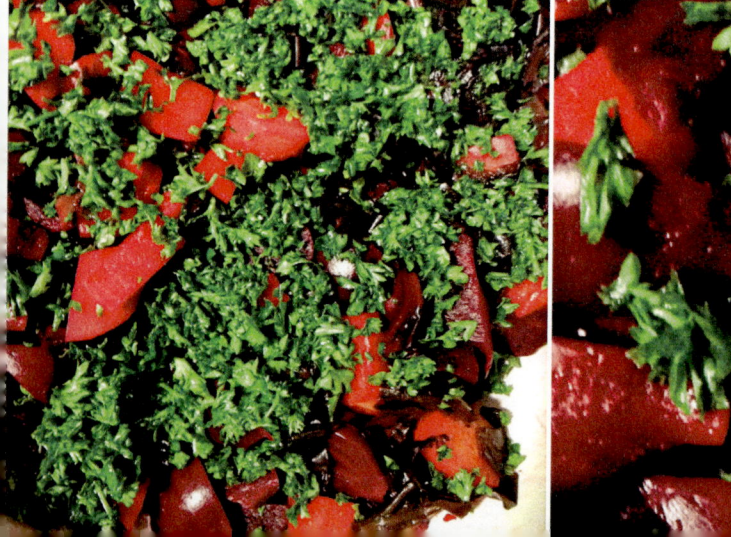
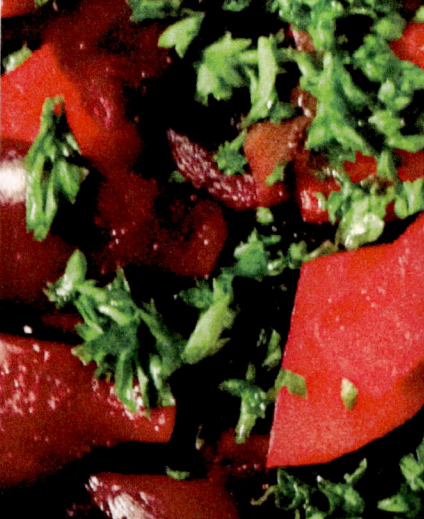

Preparation

1. Wash and quarter beets, leaving the skin on. Cook the beets. Place each batch of beets in a pot and cover with water by about an inch. Add a couple teaspoons of salt. Bring to a boil and reduce to a simmer. Simmer until you can just pierce easily with a fork, 25 to 30 minutes, depending on the size of the beets. Drain. Let cool. Rub the skins off.

2. While the beets are cooking, add the seaweed and cook for 5-8 minutes on top of beets. Remove. Let it cool, cut into 1inch pieces. Mix it all together, season with salt and pepper to taste.

3. Cut the beets into 1/2-inch to 1-inch pieces and toss with other ingredients. Chill for an hour or up to two days. *Enjoy it!*

Alkaline Forming Foods Salad

This refreshing salad has great anti-inflammatory properties! Researchers gave watercress a score of 100 for its nutritional value compared to all leafy greens. Watercress is highly alkalinizing and contains excellent minerals. Also, radicchio has been noted for its anti-cancer properties for all types of cancer!

Ingredients

2 red beets steamed, cut into bite sizes

3 to 4 radicchio leaves washed and cut into bite sizes

½ bunch of watercress or upland cress leaves washed in water vinegar as watercress carry tiny bugs-micros on the leaves

1 c. organic baby lettuces

1/2 ripe avocado smashed completely

2 -3 Inch kelp or laver seaweed washed and cooked 5 minutes

Easy alkalizing dressing:

1 cup of parsley leaves, washed and chopped

¼ c. lemon juice

1 tbs. organic flaxseed oil

¼ tsp. lemon zest

Sea Salt to taste

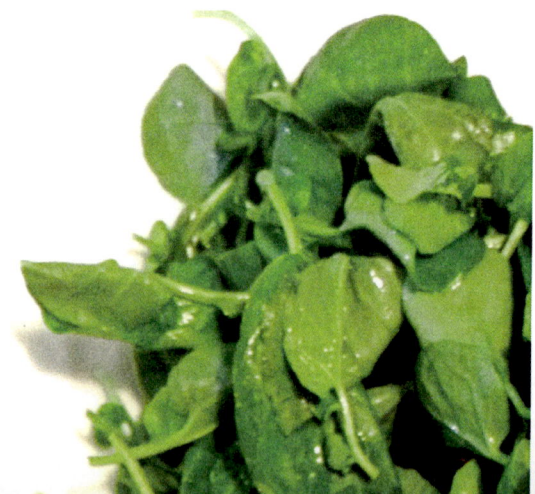
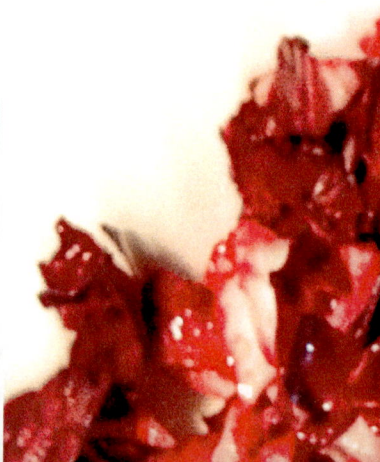

Preparation

Mix vegetable ingredients in a medium sized bowl.

For the dressing, place smashed avocado, chopped parsley leaves and lemon on separate bowl, mix them together, add flaxseed oil, salt, lemon zest, let it stand for 5 minutes. When ready to eat the salad, pour over vegetables mix them well. *Enjoy the alkalizing salad!*

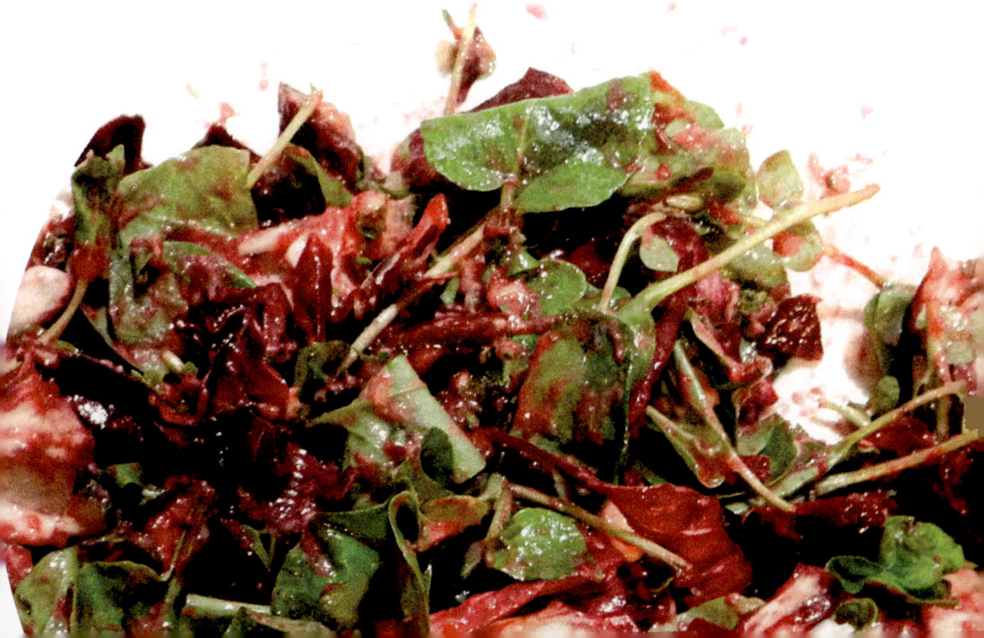

Lilly's Ground Vegetable Salad

Rich in vitamins and minerals, this colorful salad has lots of antioxidants and anti-inflammatory properties. It is also a wonderful source of fiber. Burdock is an especially fibrous root that contains inulin prebiotics , has a bitter nature, cleanses the blood, cleanses the skin and helps the liver.

Ingredients

1 medium carrot

2 big kale leaves

2-3 green cabbage leaves

1-2 celery stalk

1/2 a beet

5 inch burdock root cooked

1 cup sprouted mung beans cooked (5 minutes) 1/4 onion

1 cup cilantro or dill leaves.

2 tbs. toasted sesame oil

5-6 tbs. lemon juice

2 tbs. black sesame seeds

Salt to taste

Preparation

1. Wash all the veggies. Then cut them into medium pieces and place into a food processor. Then grind them until they are the size of rice.

2. Let the vegetables steam over boiled water for 4 minutes.

3. In a small pot, boil cook in water (boil steam) the chopped burdock root and mung beans for about 8-10 minutes.
Mix the ingredients from the two pots together, add the dressing and *enjoy!*

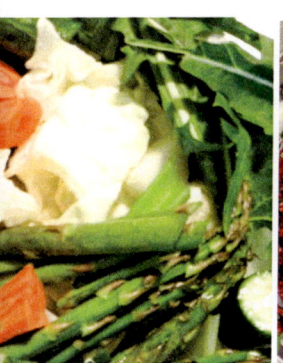
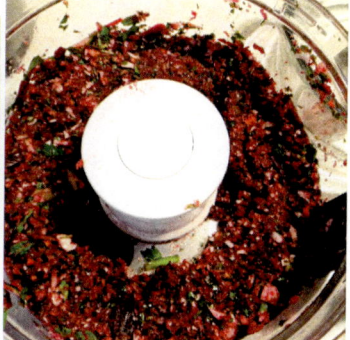
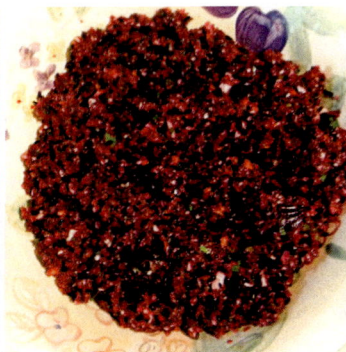

Cruciferous Veggies with Bean Fettuccini

Kale has sweet and slightly bitter, pungent flavors. It benefits the stomach and has an abundance of sulfur. It is an exceptional source of chlorophyl and minerals.Cabbage moistens the intestines and improves digestion, mental depression and irritability. It contains Vitamin U, which is a natural healer of ulcers. It is a rich source of Vitamin C and Iodine.

Ingredients

1 maitake mushroom (1bag), chopped

2 Baby bok choy washed and chopped

35 g. mung fettucini or black bean pasta

1 ½ c. red or green cabbage chopped small (packed)

1 ½ c. kale, chopped

2 clove garlic chopped

½ onion chopped

1/4 c. spring water

2 tbs. olive oil

½ c. fresh cilantro or parsley

2 tbs. fresh ginger grind or dried powder

2 tbs. fresh lemon juice

Sea Salt to taste

Preparation

In a medium size skillet of medium-low heat put water to boil, add mushrooms, garlic, ginger, onions cover let it cook for 3 minutes, add mix chopped vegetables, cover and let it cook 5 to 7 minutes according to how you like them crunchy or soft. Right before they are done stir them, add olive oil, salt. Let it stand 1 minute, uncover add lemon and cilantro and add cooked mung bean pasta in! mix all ingredients including 2 -3 tablespoons of the sauté liquid, stir several time, enjoy it! It makes a delicious, nutrient-rich meal!

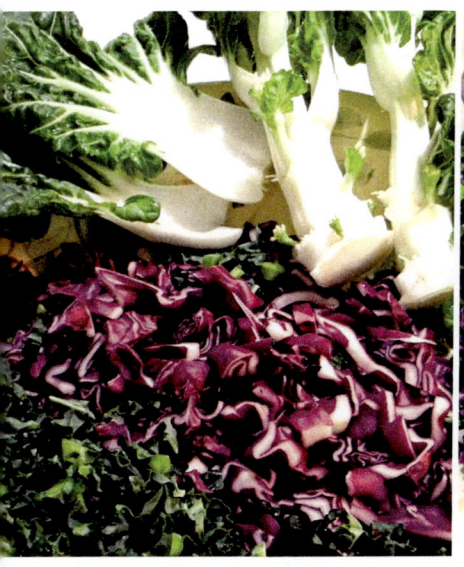 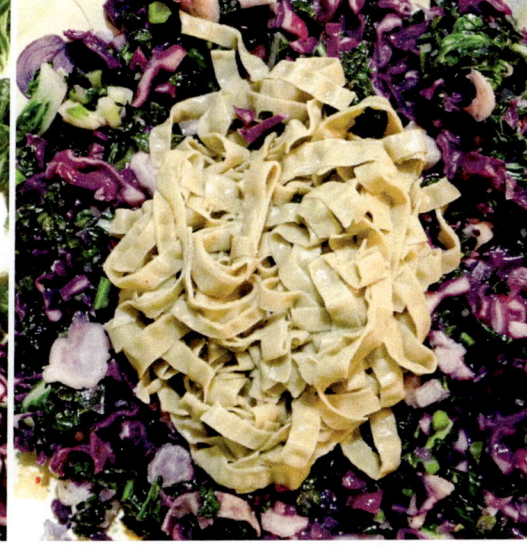

Lilly's Nutritious Garbanzo & Mushrooms Stew

This dish is a good source of protein, calcium, magnesium, folate, zinc, selenium, iron, and vitamins. Kelp seaweed alkalinizes the blood, aleviates liver stagnancy, acts as a lymphatic cleanser, and contains mucilaginous soothing gels which help the lungs and the digestive tract. Seaweed is a great source of minerals.

Ingredients

1 1/2 cup pre-cooked garbanzo beans

2 c water to warm up garbanzo beans and use as base for stew

3 big garlic cloves, minced

1 yellow onion chopped small

7 inch washed kelp seaweed, cut bite size pieces

1 cup oyster or maitake mushrooms, chopped big pieces

4 to 5 plum tomatoes, quartered – 1 stalk of celery, chopped

1 organic yellow neck squash

1 organic zucchini

1 organic red bell pepper

2 carrots, all chopped

1 tbs. coriander power

1/4 tsp. black pepper to taste

1 tbs. Sea Salt , depends on your taste for salt

1/2 cup chopped parsley leaves

1 tsp. cinnamon powder

2 tbs. olive oil

2-3 tbs. lemon juice

1/4 cup sprouted almonds, chopped

Preparation

In a large stockpot, on medium heat, put water to boil, add garlic, seaweed and onions. Let water boil for 10 minutes, add rinsed garbanzo beans and mushrooms. Let it boil for 10 minutes. Meanwhile, cut tomatoes in medium quarters, put aside. Stir in salt, coriander and cinnamon into the pot. Add all veggies, but the tomatoes, stir in and mix all together, add water if needed. Let it cook for 20 minutes, then add chopped tomatoes, cook for another 7 minutes. Add olive oil, black pepper cover, let it stand 5 minutes. Before serving add lemon juice, mix well. *Serve with chopped almonds on top! Chew well (mindfully) and enjoy the flavors!*

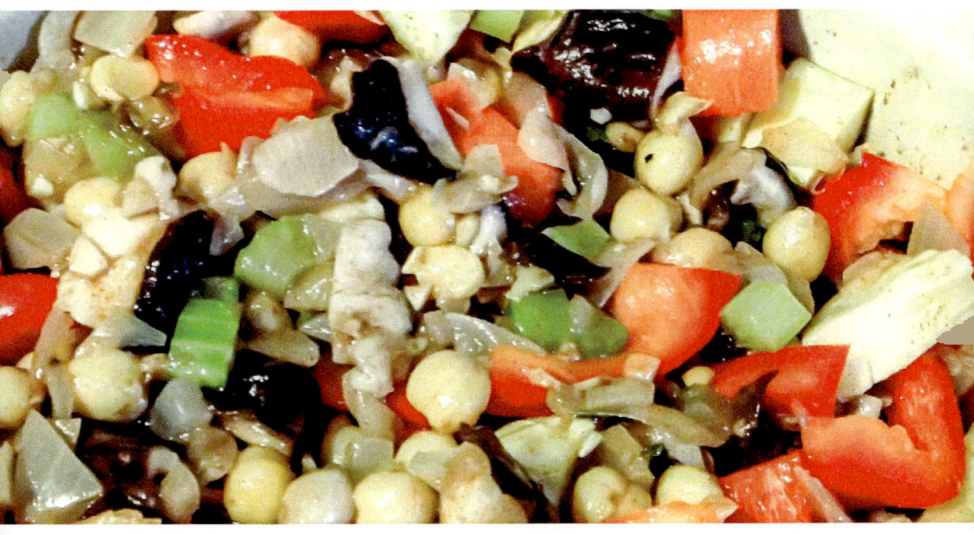

Lilly's Millet Polenta Style

Millet is more alkaline than other grains, provides good iron, protein-amino acids and minerals for good health. It is a versatile grain, makes wonderful rice-like dishes and soups. It can be used alone or mixed with other grains (oats, quinoa, amaranth). Goes really well with leafy greens!

Ingredients

4 cups water (depending on the kind of pot you are using- add ¼ c more in the last 10 minutes)
1 cup soaked organic millet (soaked overnight)
1 bunch organic cilantro, washed and chopped
7" dried kelp seaweed- rinsed, chopped or cut with scissors into tiny pieces
1 big yellow onion chopped small pieces
1 teaspoon chia seeds
¼ teaspoon turmeric
1 tsp. sea salt or salt to taste
2 1/2 tbs. olive oil

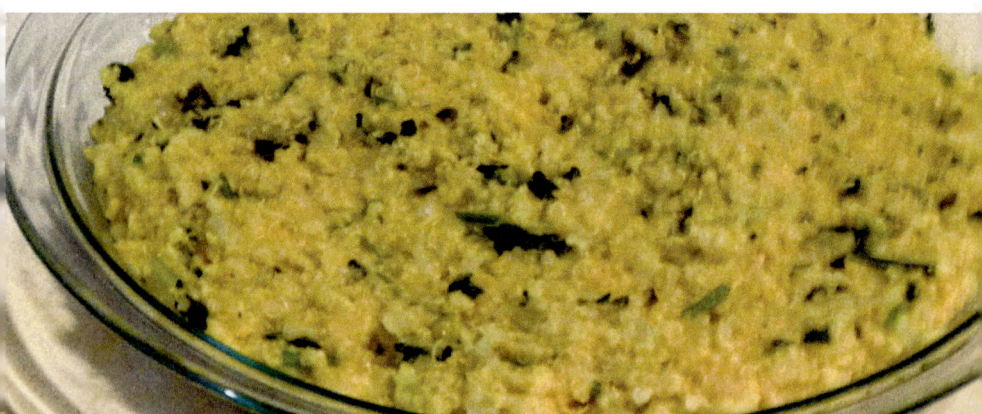

Preparation

1. Boil water in a pot, add rinsed millet. Allow to boil on high for 5 minutes, it would have foam on top, disregard foam out with spoon. Then add onions, seaweed mix well, reduce heat to medium-low, stir it, cover it and simmer for 20 to 25-minutes. Then add chopped cilantro, turmeric, olive oil, chia seeds, stir it several times. Cover it and cook for 10 minutes in low heat or until water is completely absorbed. Let it stand covered for 5-10 minutes.

2. Then transfer cooked millet into a glass container, let cool down, it would take the shape of the container, choose how thick or thin you would like it to be cut into polenta style pieces. Once it is cool millet sticks together like glue in one piece and can be cut onto solid pieces. Let it cool.

3. Let it stand for 30 minutes in the glass container until ready to be cut. You might eat it alone, or as a base for a vegetable or salad. I usually have it with my veggie pesto or sauce on top, avocado pieces and salad for a complete meal!

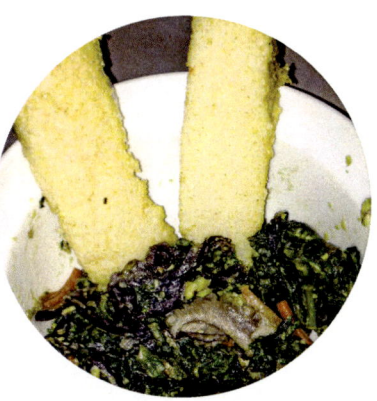

Lilly's Nutritious Whole Grain Tortillas

Simple and easy to do, the tortillas can be frozen for later use. My gluten free tortillas provide protein, good source of nutrients, fiber and are easy to digest!

Ingredients

1 c garbanzo flour

¾ c. quinoa or buckwheat flour (better to use sprouted flours if possible)

1 ½ to 1¾ c. water to mix flours, depends how thin-thick you prefer them

Himalayan salt to taste, or ½ teaspoon

1 tbs. black toasted sesame seeds

¼ tsp. turmeric powder (anti-inflammatory)

¼ tsp. cumin powder (great anti-oxidant)

¼ tsp. coconut oil to use over griddle only - spread it evenly

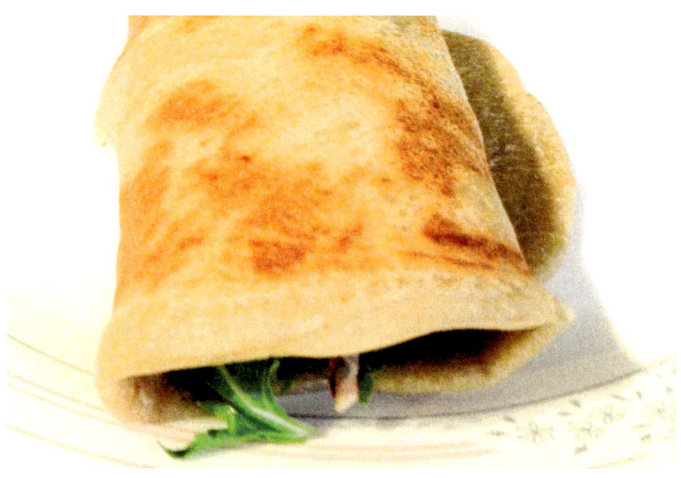

Preparation

1. In a glass bowl, mix flours with
water until soft. The batter needs
to be smooth to make the tortillas.
Add salt, let it stand for 10 minutes.
Meanwhile, warm up your griddle,
add the oil evenly over the area
where the tortilla will be cooked,

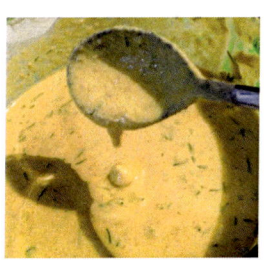

and heat the griddle until drops of water dance and evaporate
immediately. Check your batter for desired thickness. Add
spices and salt, mix until it is smooth again.

2. Spoon out the batter over the
griddle until you get the tortilla size
you desire, then spread the mix in
a circular way from the center out
to make them flat and thin. They
can be medium-sized tortillas or
large like crepes. Cook the tortilla

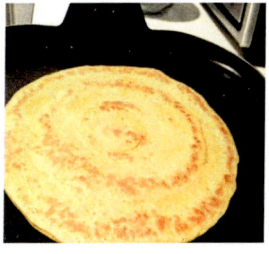

on the griddle for 5 to 7 minutes or until water evaporates and
it is crisp but not burned. Flip it over and cook the other side
for 3 minutes. Depending on how big you make them, they
can be used to wrap salads, arugula, pressed leafy greens,
or smashed avocado with sprouts! Pull it out of the griddle,
wait a minute to place in the filling veggies, then roll it up and
enjoy!

Lilly's Quick Fruitty-Coconut Dessert

Fruits are wonderful nutritious way to satisfy sweet cravings. Coconut flour is a delicious low glycemic option to make desserts creamier, chia seeds add some protein and good anti-inflammatory omega 3 fatty acids. Enjoy it!

Ingredients

1-2 hand full organic blackberries, cut in halves

1-2 kiwis, skin off, chopped small bite sizes

2 tbs. raw sprouted almonds, chopped pieces

1/2 tsp. chia seeds, mix in 1 tbs. water 5 minutes (good omega 3)

2-3 tbs. raw coconut flour (sweet-creamy delicious for desserts)

Preparation

In a medium size glass bowl mix fruits, chia seeds, coconut flour and almonds. Mix all ingredients until fruits looks creamy, cover it, let it stand 10 minutes. It is ready to eat! Enjoy this refreshing, nutritious light dessert.

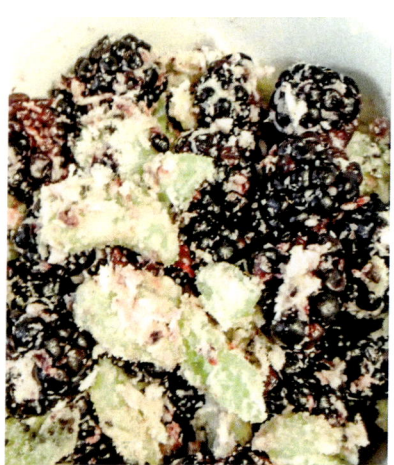

Eating With A Purpose In Mind

Both Eastern and Western nutrition agree in the anti-cancer and anti-inflammatory properties of these groups of foods. I have been using these foods to create food synergy in my recipes. Matching, mixing and eating consistently these foods had helped me, and my clients to send the right message to the cells. Start slowly building up the habit, and adjusting your taste buds to the new foods. I certainly love guiding my clients into building a delicious, nutritious menu with strong immunity and anti-cancer properties that suits their unique lifestyle and needs.

Here are the top anti-inflammatory, anti-cancer food groups that I have been using:

Cruciferous Vegetables:

- Arugula
- Bok choy
- Broccoli
- Broccoli sprouts
- Brussels sprouts
- Cabbage
- Cauliflower
- Chinese cabbage
- Collard greens
- Daikon radish
- Horseradish
- Kale
- Kohlrabi
- Mustard greens
- Radish
- Rutabaga
- Turnip
- Watercress

This vegetable group is the highest in vitamin A carotenoids, vitamin C, folic acid, minerals, fiber and anti-oxidants. Cruciferous vegetables are a nutritional powerhouse. They are high in vitamin K content, which helps regulate inflammatory responses, including chronic inflammation that increases the risk of cancers.

Mushrooms:

- Shitake
- Maitake

Mushrooms are a good source of germanium, which improves cellular oxygenation and enhances immunity. These mushrooms are a natural source of interferon, a protein which appears to induce an immune response against cancer and viral diseases. Also, oyster mushrooms have been in many studies, as they help regulate blood sugar, used for diabetes and inflammatory diseases. A study published in the international Journal of Cancer showed women who regularly consumed mushrooms are 64% less likely to develop breast cancer.

Seaweed Kelp:

General Properties of Seaweeds: a cooling thermal nature; salty flavor; soften hardened areas and masses in the body; detoxify; moisten dryness; transform phlegm; diuretic; remove residues of radiation in the body; build the yin fluids and improve water metabolism; act as lymphatic cleansers; alkalize the blood; alleviate liver stagnancy (activate liver qi); beneficial to the thyroid. Seaweeds are useful in weight-loss programs and for lowering cholesterol and fat in the blood.

From the TCM traditional food therapy, marine plants have a "sinking" quality and hence direct the energy of the body lower and more internally. Seaweeds in general are used to treat swellings, nodules, lumps, goiter, swollen lymph glands, edema, chronic heat signs such as yellow or green phlegm, all skin diseases marked with redness, and tumors. They are also useful in cancer and fibroid tumors. According to ancient Chinese believes, "there is no swelling that is not relieved by seaweed."

Onions:

Onions are make up the allium family of vegetables. They provide us with a powerful content of polyphenols and anti-cancer properties.

- Garlic
- Chives
- Onions
- Leeks
- Shallots

Other Foods That Possess Cancer-Inhibiting Properties :

- Leafy greens and algaes such as: spirulina, chlorella, and wheat-barley grasses.
- Celery
- Parsley
- Carrots
- Asparagus
- Turmeric
- Ginger
- Daikon Radish
- Berries, such as: blueberries, raspberries, mulberries, blackberries,
- Lemon
- Tomatoes
- Green tea
- Okra
- Grapefruit
- Sea cucumber

Sprouts, specially broccoli sprouts have been in many studies for their powerful properties against breast cancer.

Forming Habits
And Adapting To A Better Health

The easiest way to really eat healthier foods is to form healthy habits. We are meant to function in habitual routines. Most of the time we shop for the same foods, go around the store in the same circles and prepare the same type of dishes at home or go to our favorite restaurants. These are some of the habits we have. If we keep eating the same foods, we will get the same results in our energy and health states, since the food we eat impacts the chemistry of our bodies. But you have the power to change your chemistry.

In order to increase nutrition, immunity and avoid diseases, we need to change and prioritize our nutritional habits, lifestyles, shopping lists, and cooking habits. I have seen it again and again with my clients, my family and myself. I would have probably not survived cancer without changing my nutritional habits and lifestyle. Introducing nutritionally dense foods and creating easy steps to make them into a lifestyle habit was probably the best thing that has happened to me. Now it is second nature to eat healthy, whole, and powerful foods, both for me and for my clients. That's what really works - sending the right message to your cells consistently. I love helping my clients achieve this. First they become aware of their habits, then I introduce new dense specific needs and guide them to form effortless habits that work for their health and happiness. What habits are not serving you at this time? What would help you to move forward in creating the habits that you need for good health? Would having support be beneficial to you? It is all about creating the right habits and priorities!

Conclusion: The Big Picture and The Circle of Health

Since everything in life moves in a circular spiral manner, from our DNA to the milky way in the galaxies; from our atoms, cells and systems in our body to the daily day and night routine; from the way plants open up their leaves in nature to the way cyclones and ocean currents move. Everything is consistently circulating and vibrating. Wouldn't it be helpful for our health to be in sync with life's natural circulating rhythmic patterns and allow our habits, routines and bio-rhythms to circulate, from start to finish, with this natural pattern as well?

*This holistic **circle of health** is a way for promoting an easy natural flow for our digestive system, liver, blood, kidneys, lungs, heart, and all body systems, especially our immune system, to work efficiently against cancer. After all, our systems are meant to be circulating! So avoiding stagnation in any tissue, organ or system, promoting **consistent rhythmic circulation** of energy, blood, and toxic waste, makes sense. Which routines in your life can you improve or create to avoid stagnation in your body and life?*

I would love to hear from you and listen to your stories! Feel free to connect with me:
website: www.lillypadilla.com ,
e-mail: lpadillacreate@gmail.com
Facebook page: lillypadilla holistichealth

I hope you join my online community! Health and harmony to you! - Lilly

TESTIMONIALS

"My entire relationship with food has shifted for the better since working with Lilly. I always considered myself a healthy eater but when I received a cancer diagnosis in 2011 I knew I needed to take a look at my diet. I have always been a busy person with no time to cook. In fact I have NEVER liked cooking and used the microwave quite a bit. Since working with Lilly I have come to LOVE cooking, love my kitchen and food shopping! She is incredible! She makes food FUN and most of my life that was not the case. Lilly helped me to create a food plan personalized for me and for my health needs. We have cooked and shopped together so I no longer feel overwhelmed by all of the choices in the markets. I make weekly trips to the Farmer's Market with confidence on how to purchase the freshest products. I have learned how to shop what is in season and prepare healthy meals very quickly almost every day of the week. Lilly provides tips on how to prepare foods quickly so if I don't have a lot of time or come home from a long day - cooking is fast, easy and healthy! I haven't worried about gaining weight for

the first time in 30 years! My energy has increased and sugar cravings have decreased. I am also getting more organized and feeling more balanced in my life. I technically have "graduated" from Lilly's program but I will continue to meet with her as needed and will be forever grateful to her for her inspiration. She is truly an angel & I am blessed to have her in my life!"

- Sharon H.

Within two months of working with Lilly I have lost 12 lbs and my cholesterol numbers have dropped dramatically. I began to eat whole foods rather than the easy pre packaged meals or fast foods I gravitated toward. I feel great, sleep better, and have more energy. With Lilly's caring, support, and knowledge, she has taught me how to make smart choices for my body when it comes to shopping for groceries, preparing food, dinning out, and how I will eat the rest of my life. She really gave me the encouragement and confidence to change my life style. I recently had a follow-up visit with my cardiologist and he was very pleasantly surprised with my test results. The words of my cardiologist... "Congratulations regarding your outstanding initial response to significant lifestyle changes that have resulted in a dramatic reduction in your cholesterol and markedly reduced triglyceride level. Keep up the great work!" I would recommend Lilly and her experience to anyone who wants to change their life, and I look forward to continuing to work with her. This is one of the best investments I have ever made"

- Yvonne L.

Aknowledgements

Special thanks to all my clients, fans, cancer survivors and to Joshua Rosenthal for motivating me to write this book. My clients' encouragement and requests for this book kept me moving forward. Thanks to the many people who provided help, love and support. Writing this book has been a wonderful, challenging and exciting experience.

I'm deeply appreciative to Nicole Leibman, my designer and main editor, thank you for your tireless, great work on this book. And special thanks to Yang-chu for sharing his knowledge of Traditional Chinese Medicine. Also, I would like to thank Dr. Sonia Warren for her support and encouragement. I'm also grateful to Doctor Albert Marti Bosch whose expertise as a Holistic Oncologist opened up a door for understanding cancer from a different perspective.

I would like to also thank my Mother, brothers and sisters for their love, and support, and my father for teaching me to love nature, work and life, and Paco, my rescue dog companion, who rescued me, and took me for walks when I was weak and sick, I love you. A special thanks goes to Ilena, Kathy, Grasiela, Rose, Elizabeth, Diana and Hector for your support and editing help.

Thanks to all my teachers, without you I wouldn't have changed my lifestyle, nutrition and improved my life. Finally, thanks to everyone that ever wanted to improve your health and life, but didn't know how, everything I do, I do it for you.

Bibliography

Brones, Anna. "Does Dirt Make You Happy?." Well Being Journal Jul.-Aug. 2015. Print.

Liponis, Mark. *Ultra-Longevity: The Seven-Step Program For a Younger, Healthier You.* New York: Little, Brown, 2007. Print.

Lupien, Sonia. Well Stressed: How You Can Manage Stress Before It Turns Toxic. Ont.:John Wiley & Sons, 2012. Print.

Matveikova, Irina, Dr. "Digestive Intelligence: Microflora, Gut Health, and Your Second Brain." Well Being Journal Jan.-Feb. 2015. Print.

Ni, Maoshing. *The Yellow Emperor's Classic of Medicine: A New Translation of the Neijing Suwen with Commentary.* Boston: Shambhala, 1995. Print

"7 Million Premature Deaths Annually Linked to Air Pollution." WHO. N.p., 25 Mar. 2014. Web.

World Association Cancer Research - Dr. Alberto Marti Bosch. YoutTube. Blogsaludconsciente, 18

Jan. 2013. Web.
Genetic Roulette - The Gamble of Our Lives. Dir. Jeffrey Smith. 2012.

Quantum Healing Update. By Deepak Chopra. YouTube. N.p., 27 Jan. 2015. Web.

Made in the USA
San Bernardino, CA
10 August 2019